HOLISTIC
PAIN RELIEF

Praise for *Holistic Pain Relief*

"Thank heaven for Dr. Tick's *Holistic Pain Relief*. As a physician who has practiced and taught emergency medicine for over thirty years, I frequently encounter people in pain, both acute and chronic, and have often been stymied as to how to help — until now. Dr. Tick's thorough and humane approach to the evaluation and unique comprehensive management of pain is truly a breakthrough. It should be read and embraced by all practitioners of the healing arts."

— Peter W. Rugg, MD, FACEP, past chair, department of emergency medicine, UMass Memorial HealthAlliance Hospital

"Very well done and a pleasure to read, *Holistic Pain Relief* is a truly helpful example of a self-help book, packed with much more information than the average of the genre."

— John D. Loeser, MD, professor of neurosurgery, University of Washington, and former president, International Association for the Study of Pain

"Dr. Heather Tick has provided a valuable resource for the many people suffering from acute and chronic pain and for all of us who desire a 'whole person' approach to optimal well-being — as well as for those health care practitioners interested in a more complete understanding of the use of complementary and alternative medicine or integrative medicine in the context of pain. Her humanism, optimism, and profound commitment to improving the lives of pain sufferers and those under profound stress speak from every page."

— Eric B. Schoomaker, MD, PhD, Lieutenant General, US Army (retired), former Army Surgeon General, and Audrey N. Schoomaker, RN, BSN, E-RYT 500, yoga therapist

"This is a rare book on pain that is comprehensive and accessible yet scientifically grounded. The book is uniquely comprehensible and reassuring to the reader. Dr. Tick is remarkable in her ability to identify what is important and practical and to translate that information for the public."

— Ping Ho, MA, MPH, founding director, Arts and Healing Initiative, UCLA

HOLISTIC
PAIN RELIEF

DR. TICK'S BREAKTHROUGH STRATEGIES
TO MANAGE AND ELIMINATE PAIN

HEATHER TICK, MD

New World Library
Novato, California

New World Library
14 Pamaron Way
Novato, California 94949

The material in this book is intended for education. It is not meant to take the place
of diagnosis and treatment by a qualified medical practitioner or therapist. No
expressed or implied guarantee of the effects of the use of the recommendations can
be given nor liability taken.

Text design by Tona Pearce Myers

Library of Congress Cataloging-in-Publication Data
Tick, Heather, date.
Holistic pain relief : Dr. Tick's breakthrough strategies to manage and eliminate
pain / Heather Tick, MD.
    pages   cm
Includes bibliographical references and index.
ISBN 978-1-60868-206-5 (pbk.) — ISBN 978-1-60868-207-2 (ebook)
 1. Pain—Alternative treatment—Popular works. 2. Pain—Treatment—Popular
works. 3. Holistic medicine. I. Title.
RB127.T53 2013
616'.0472—dc23   2013028452

First printing, November 2013
ISBN 978-1-60868-206-5
Printed in the USA on 100% postconsumer-waste recycled paper

New World Library is proud to be a Gold Certified Environmentally
Responsible Publisher. Publisher certification awarded by Green Press
Initiative. www.greenpressinitiative.org

10 9 8 7 6 5 4 3 2 1

To my children, Noah, Emma, and Seth:
I admire your commitment and ideals, your grace, courage, and joyfulness.
You have brought love and beauty into my life.
With gratitude for your unwavering support.

CONTENTS

Part I. Breaking New Ground

Part II. Pain Solutions

Part III. The Next Steps

PART I

BREAKING NEW GROUND

CHAPTER I

PAIN, NATURE'S WAKE-UP CALL

*The merest schoolgirl when she falls in love has Shakespeare or Keats
to speak her mind for her, but let a sufferer try to describe
a pain in his head to a doctor and language at once runs dry.*

— VIRGINIA WOOLF, *On Being Ill*

For me, questions about pain and its treatment started during my first year of medical school at the University of Toronto. One day I noticed that I was experiencing a strange, nagging pain in my right shoulder. Like most of us who suddenly realize that Pain, the Intruder, has arrived on our doorstep, I fully expected it to go away on its own.

It was there the next day, and the day after. Although I tried to ignore it, that was impossible when I lifted my arm to reach overhead. I'd be jolted back to the reality that this pain wasn't going anywhere by itself. Instead, the pain was growing sharper, and if I maneuvered something heavy overhead, it felt even worse.

Over the course of three weeks, putting my arm behind me to pull

3

on a sweater or coat became harder and harder, but I kept doing it to stretch the muscles and not lose the function. For the life of me, I couldn't remember what I'd done to cause this, so I continued to hope it would go away as silently as it had come.

I was still in my twenties with a pretty healthy diet and a regular exercise routine, so I told myself there was nothing to worry about. But then, a month passed, and I now had difficulty raising my arm above shoulder height. Finding a comfortable position to sleep proved trying. I was in pain when cooking meals that required extensive stirring and chopping. Carrying my schoolbooks hurt.

Finally, I accepted the inevitable: time to get some over-the-counter medications. Unfortunately (or fortunately, as I will explain), they disagreed with my stomach, so I had to stop them. The pain continued for another three months. Now, I had to limit my exercise to walking, because anything I did with my arms aggravated my painful shoulder. To compensate for the lack of sleep, I drank more coffee to stay awake in classes. A cloud of unhappiness settled over me. All I could think about was my shoulder; it dominated every daily activity. All I wanted was to get my life back and to forget about that shoulder.

As luck would have it, I was enrolled in an evening course on acupuncture, which was not part of the regular medical school curriculum. It was offered by a group of doctors who had established the Acupuncture Foundation of Canada to train physicians to use acupuncture techniques. I listened with fascination as one doctor lectured about theories of why it worked and why the Chinese had been using it for thousands of years. During another class, the lecturing physician described how painful sports injuries were treated using nothing more than a very thin needle containing no medication.

One evening, two doctors showed up to lecture. It was time to demonstrate what the instructor had been lecturing on for the past four weeks. They asked for volunteers to demonstrate on, and I quickly shot up my arm — my good arm. I walked up to the front of the room, wondering if little needles might be the answer to my problem. The doctors asked me questions about the location of my shoulder pain and had me move my head and arm this way and that. One of the doctors put some alcohol on a cotton ball and swabbed my skin in about six places around my shoulder. He then took a tiny needle and, with a quick tap, pushed it into the first freshly swabbed spot. I didn't feel anything but the pressure of the tap. He inserted five other needles with the same type of quick tap. Two of the needles stung slightly when inserted. I could feel the area around the needles grow warm, but they did not cause major discomfort. After ten minutes, he removed the needles. "That's it?" I thought.

I was sent home with homework: to continue treatments on myself every other day until symptoms abated.[1] In a previous class we had learned how to insert the needles, so I was able to do acupuncture on myself using the same points that had been used in class. Within three days of my first treatment, all my symptoms had vanished. I could lift my arm pain-free, I could sleep through the night, and I could start light resistance exercises to strengthen my arm. It took another week until I regained the full range of motion in that arm.

And the best part? The problem didn't return.

Later that same year, my father developed neck and shoulder pain. His regular doctor recommended medication that proved ineffective after two weeks. The doctor had no other remedies to offer. I suggested that my father stop taking the ineffective pills, and I sent him to a chiropractor who included acupuncture in his treatments. My father was skeptical. He was convinced that the spinal adjustments would not work and ridiculed the idea that needles could remove pain. He went only to humor me. But with the combination of chiropractic care and acupuncture, my father recovered fully in six weeks. He was so impressed that he became a lifelong fan of both treatments. I found myself growing more and more fascinated by these practices that enhance the body's own ability to heal itself, with very little risk of side effects. I have been interested in pain management and alternative therapies ever since.

Throughout my practice, I have found it useful to return to the first principles: anatomy, physiology, and pathology. These are the basics that

form the foundation of medicine, and the terms refer to the body structure, the science of how our bodies work, and what we know about how
things go wrong. I am grateful that while I attended the University of
Toronto Medical School my instructors spent a long time teaching these
fundamentals. They gave me the tools to think about some of the basic
mechanisms behind people's pain, the ways pain was commonly treated,
and what happened when treatments failed. I became a family doctor
and saw patients with lingering pain that often disabled them. Some of
these people would not get better despite physical therapy, appointments
with specialists, and the use of medications. For these unfortunate sufferers, I kept looking for answers. This led me farther and farther into the
alternative fields of medicine: nutrition, massage therapy, craniosacral
therapy, acupuncture, chiropractic, and others.

I became familiar with the term *myofascial disorder*. *Myo* means
"muscle," and the fascia is the supporting tissue around the muscles. I
had gone through my entire medical education, internship, and residency
and had never heard the word until a few years after I started my practice.
As I began to read more about it, it became apparent that this was a glar-
ing omission: myofascial disorders are the most common cause of pain.[2]

I read the early works of Janet Travell, MD, who was the grandmother of myofascial therapies in the United States and served as the
physician for John F. Kennedy while he was in the White House. Then I
read the references listed in her book and was astounded at the richness of
this literature. I was introduced to the work of Dr. C. Chan Gunn, who
developed coherent theories to explain the physiology of myofascial pain
and its treatment. The writings of Janet Travell and Chan Gunn trans-
formed my vision of healing, and the treatment developed by Dr. Gunn,
called Gunn intramuscular stimulation, is the most effective tool I have
found for myofascial pain. I learned that certain common and disabling
types of chronic pain can go away with the right treatment. I have treated
over five thousand new patients and seen the results. But while these techniques solved many of my own pain problems and those of my patients,
over the years I have seen an increasing number of people with severe

pain, complex and puzzling problems, and unexplained illness associated with their pain syndromes. We have a long way to go to tackle the challenges that face us.

Since I began to practice medicine in 1984, I have seen pain as a growing problem. There are an increasing number of sufferers, including younger people developing pain syndromes, and an increase in the severity and complexity of pain problems. I even have many teenagers in my practice now who have too much pain and disability to attend school. These are normal kids, including some high-level athletes, who want desperately to get on with their lives. Complicated procedures and sophisticated drugs have limited effects — their side effects are sometimes as much a burden as the original problem. What has never been adequately studied is the resulting loss of human potential — the gifts these people have been unable to develop that could have enriched our society. This is especially the case with very young sufferers.

Everyone knows what pain is. Most of us have known pain in our own bodies and have seen it in others. But when we really try to describe what pain is, we are often at a loss for words.

Pain itself does not have an emotional component. If you pinch yourself until it hurts, you are unlikely to react with happiness, anger, fear, or sadness. An emotional reaction usually occurs only when your pain seems to be incomprehensible or out of control, when you do not know how or when it will end.

There are words for pain in every language. There is no nation or culture that is spared the experience.[3] Yet the experience of pain is a solitary one. Those who are living with pain pay in immediate suffering and by not being able to live their lives fully. Those in pain feel alone, isolated in their agony, and separated from their former lives and the lives of those around them. Pain sufferers may also feel the separation that comes with the judgments of others.

People in pain often do not "look" as though they are in pain. If they focus on their pain in conversation, or reveal their discomfort by their actions, they risk being labeled as "complainers" or "symptom magnifiers." Animals in pain instinctively seek privacy to lick their wounds. Similarly, there may be a natural instinct in people to seek comfort in withdrawal.

Pain is always a subjective experience. We have no ways to measure pain "objectively." There are charts, scales, body diagrams, and ratings, but none of them measure pain the way a thermometer measures a fever. In the end, the person in pain tells us about his pain. Patients with lingering pain almost universally have their experience of pain questioned, challenged, and disbelieved by health care practitioners and by friends and family. Most of these patients also say that the vocabulary available and the scorecards used in pain clinics do not help them convey the true experience of their pain.

Pain is complex. The issues involved spread out like the ripples from a pebble tossed into a pond. When these ripples become intermingled with the wave patterns of countless other pebbles, it becomes impossible to distinguish one pattern from the next. Chronic pain is like a fifty-thousand-piece jigsaw puzzle for which we have placed about five hundred pieces. We are not even sure what the big picture is. This is small comfort for those in pain. The good news is that, despite the lack of clarity in our vision, we have many useful interventions.

Acute pain is pain lasting a relatively short time and is usually injury related. Chronic pain is pain lasting longer than three months — or six months, depending on whose definition is used. But these are simplistic definitions of complex problems. In some cases, acute pain lasts more than six months because there has been neither an accurate diagnosis nor an appropriate treatment. In other cases, we are in the first month of a process which is already evolving into a chronic state. Nothing magical happens during the third or sixth month that makes the process different. Sometimes the pain is chronic pain from the beginning; we just didn't know. Other times, something does change in the way the body processes pain, but that may happen on day one, or day one hundred, or day three hundred. No expert can impose a timeline on Mother Nature.

The number of people who suffer from pain is staggering. That is why, in late 2000, the United States Congress passed a provision into law, signed by President Clinton, that declared the ten-year period beginning January 1, 2001, the Decade of Pain Control and Research. Countless studies have been undertaken to try to measure the effects of pain and the number of people affected. The definitions used and the variables measured are not identical from study to study, and so drawing information from them can be a little confusing. However, a decade later, the 2011 report of the Institute of Medicine, an organization in the United States that provides national advice on health issues, estimated that there were over 100 million Americans in pain.[4] This figure did not include children in pain or any individuals in acute pain. There are a lot of people in pain. And this is not just an American problem. The International Association for the Study of Pain estimates that 20 percent of adults have moderate to severe chronic pain. Professor Harald Breivik, coeditor of *Clinical Pain Management*, has called chronic pain "one of the most underestimated health care problems in the world today, causing major consequences for the quality of life of the sufferer and a major burden on the health care system in the Western world."[5]

Let us look at some of these statistics relating to costs. To begin with, pain has a cost to society, starting with costs for health care services, medication, surgery, and the complications that arise as a result of all those things. Then, there is the cost in lost productivity and absence from the workplace, which has impacts on industry but also on social service budgets and even tax revenues. The 2011 report by the Institute of Medicine estimated the annual cost of chronic pain in the United States at between $560 and $635 billion.[6] The report called for a "culture change" in the medical system that treats pain.

In 2004 Americans spent $16.6 billion to relieve pain, most of it to purchase over-the-counter or prescription drugs.[7] Pain is a problem for insurance companies too. The costs of high-tech procedures and surgeries like epidural injections, spinal cord stimulators and pumps, and spinal surgeries are rising each year. And what is worse is that we seem to be setting people up for other problems down the line. We are spending more and more and not getting people better.

When we look at the workplace, some costs of pain are easier to quantify than others. We can get the annual statistics for Workers' Compensation costs and lost workdays. What are harder to assess are the costs associated with people in pain who come to work but are unable to work at their full capacity, a phenomenon called "presenteeism."

A survey done by Gallup in 2011 found that nearly 47 percent of adults reported having a condition affecting the neck, the back, a lower limb, or another part of the body that caused recurring pain in the previous twelve months.[8] Low-income Americans are even more likely to have chronic pain. Nearly 50 percent of all Americans seek care for pain each year.[9]

No matter how you measure it, pain is a big problem: for the person in pain, for those providing treatment, for the insurer who is paying for treatment and time off work, for the employer waiting for an employee to return to work, for the kids who want their parent to play catch, and for other family members living with the person in pain. Unfortunately, conventional approaches to the treatment of pain often do not improve the situation.

Though most physicians would prefer to treat each patient as a unique case, many now adhere to practice guidelines — established signposts intended to shape the problem-solving path followed by physicians. Practice guidelines were originally designed as a sound basis for the minimum care a physician should offer but are now used as welcome assistance to the rushed physician who can spend only a few minutes with each patient.

Recent studies of patient-physician visits show that primary-care physicians in North America spend an average of 10.7 minutes with each patient.[10] The doctors studied allowed the patient to speak for only eighteen seconds before they interrupted.[11] This leaves very little time for nuanced communication and attention to the complexities that characterize most human conditions. There is barely time to decide which drug to prescribe before drawing the meeting to a close.

Physicians may also feel pressure to follow the standard-of-care practices — to do what most others in the community are doing. For example, prescribing the anti-inflammatory drug Vioxx was the standard of care for many years, even though evidence, little known to most doctors, indicated that it increased the risk of heart attack. Few doctors read the studies to learn about the drug's risk; instead, they simply looked at the information the drug reps handed them. When I presented information about this risk to a group of colleagues two years before Vioxx was pulled from the market, I was called an alarmist. Most of my colleagues continued prescribing the drug until it was no longer available. These are issues that I explore in greater detail in the pages that follow.

I have written this book as a patients' guide to understanding and managing chronic pain. Chronic pain is a growing problem, one that affects more people than before, with increasing severity; and now there are new types of pain that are unresponsive to conventional therapies. There is a growing body of scientific literature explaining the mechanisms of pain and how we experience it. But despite more research and knowledge, there are still patients with confusing collections of symptoms that defy explanation. For these people, chronic pain is just one piece of a complex puzzle that is the healthy human body.

The fact is, we pain physicians don't have all the answers, and we know it. Being a pain doctor takes courage — the courage to travel the path with our patients, to be present as they present us with their vulnerabilities and look to us for answers that we may not have. It takes courage to tell patients when we don't have the answers, and it is our responsibility to tell them with kindness, without blaming them for defeating our knowledge, and without making them feel abandoned. *Cor*, Latin for "heart," is the root word for *courage*. Most pain physicians practice because they care. There are two vulnerable people in the room during a pain visit: the patient and the doctor.

My goal is always to treat people with compassion, to ease their suffering, and to reassure them that their voices are heard.

CHAPTER 2

THE CHANGING TIMES

As to diseases, make a habit of two things — to help,
or at least, to do no harm.

— HIPPOCRATES, *Epidemics*

A s it stands, the American health care system is the most expensive in the world. Yet what do we have to show for it? The United States ranks approximately fiftieth in the world for life expectancy.[1] A study published by the *Journal of the American Medical Association* in 2000 concluded that our health care system itself is the third-leading cause of death in the country. This study took into account only hospitalized patients, but it covered a host of causes, including errors, unnecessary surgeries, infections, and the side effects of properly prescribed drugs approved by the Food and Drug Administration.[2] The study estimated that there are 225,000 patient deaths per year. Only the fast-food and cigarette industries can compete.[3] In our current health care system, there is very little care and almost no attention to health. I would go so far as to say that we don't have a health care system; we have an illness-management system. How did it come to this?

In 1908, there were around 160 medical schools in the United States and Canada. They were a mix of university-based medical schools and alternative ones. Alternative schools included those that taught homeopathy, chiropractic, naturopathy, and folk medicine. That year, the American Medical Association and the Carnegie Foundation commissioned Abraham Flexner to write a report setting needed standards for medical education. Flexner, however, was an educator with no medical background. He was used to the more regimented, European-style education of the university-based schools. He criticized the alternative schools for being unscientific. As a result of his report, the diversity of medical education in the United States and Canada was drastically reduced. By 1930, of the previously mentioned 160 medical schools, only 76 remained. Needless to say, almost all of the remaining schools were university based.

Medical doctors became the main authorities on the practice of medicine, holding a virtual monopoly. Osteopathy, naturopathy, and other alternative systems of education and treatment were discredited; at the same time, medical education became less available to women, people of color, and low-income applicants. The regimented, university-based medical education taught allopathic medicine, which became the dominant form of practice in North America for over a hundred years. (Allopathic medicine is what we call the conventional practices of medical doctors today.) In 2011, Thomas Duffy, MD, published an article analyzing the Flexner report. In his article, Duffy writes, "After Flexner, medicine lost its soul."[4]

Flexner was right: allopathic medicine is more regimented than the alternatives. But that doesn't mean it's more scientific. The majority of both allopathic and alternative methods are supported by very little evidence that is considered adequate. The major difference between the two is the risks involved in practicing each. In the words of Hippocrates, often regarded as the father of Western medicine, we should, first, "do no harm." Remember the 225,000 patient deaths per year? Our current health care system, an allopathic one, constantly causes harm. Despite this, we have supported it for a hundred years.

Allopathic medicine is more regimented than the alternatives because it is problem focused, not person focused. Whether an appointment with a primary-care practitioner, a visit with a specialist, or a trip to urgent care or the emergency department, the vast majority of medical encounters are initiated because of a problem, usually one having to do with pain. When you see a doctor, you are asked why you are there. What is the problem that made you think you needed a doctor? The entire visit is dominated by the need for the doctor to chart the problem. We chart problems to understand them but also to get paid for seeing you — obviously, we do need to get paid. You are asked many questions about the problem. How did it start? What does it feel like? What makes it better or worse? The doctor's charting is designed to capture the details of the problem. Over the years, our notes required by insurance companies have gotten more and more detailed. Sometimes, it seems we spend more time looking after the notes about the patients than looking after the patients themselves.

By the end of the visit, we are expected to come up with an assessment of the problem and then a treatment plan for the problem. If we connect with the patient as a human being, that is not important to the insurance company paying for the visit; it's a bonus. But given the rushed schedules and the push for us to see more patients in less time, it's a rarity. Patients sometimes feel as though they get lost in the system. Sometimes they do. Patients who want to stay healthy have a difficult time finding the guidance they need to do so, because the system is meant to engage with them only once they have a problem.

Doctors get paid very little to spend time talking to patients, trying to figure out all the complicated details of what is really going on. Doctors do not get paid for good outcomes, either. There isn't even a way of measuring whether we are keeping our patients healthy. On the other hand, our system pays doctors well for seeing large numbers of patients and for doing procedures. It's piecework. In hospitals, doctors get quotas and bonuses for seeing more patients. In private clinics, seeing more patients means higher incomes. Doctors become anxious to diagnose quickly so they can move on to the next patient on their tight schedules. The focus is less and less on the whole person and more on the specific problems, each of which has a specific answer.

The child with an ear infection gets a quick prescription for an antibiotic. The young woman with high cholesterol gets cholesterol-lowering medication. In the child's case, the doctor may have noticed that this is his fifth ear infection of the year but does not dig deeper into the possible underlying causes — a poor diet leading to a weak immune system or an allergy to cow's milk leading to mucus congestion. During a follow-up visit with the young woman, the doctor sees that the patient's cholesterol levels are now lower and so repeats the prescription. The young woman may have muscle aches but does not know they could be from the cholesterol drug, and the doctor, focused only on the numbers associated with the problem — the high cholesterol — does not ask.

Allopathic medicine compartmentalizes people. Medical textbooks are written that way, and the emphasis on medical specialties encourages this approach. The way diseases are named, the way procedures are developed, even the way medical research is funded, all further this idea: a person is a collection of parts, and a disease is just a malfunction of one part alone. But a patient is more than just "the rotator cuff in exam room 3."

The second half of the twentieth century saw an acceleration in the development of medical specialties. As medical knowledge expanded rapidly, there were good reasons to have specialists with intensive understandings in specific areas. But there were also economic factors that led physicians to be specialists instead of primary-care doctors: specialists earn a lot more. Currently, in the United States, graduating medical students choose specialty training three times more often than they choose primary care. Primary-care training programs fill 45 percent of their spaces with US graduates, while many specialty programs fill over 90 percent with US grads.

There are some problems with this. Demand for specific procedures in a region should correlate to the needs of the patients in that region. What we find, however, is a higher demand for certain procedures in regions that have a higher supply of doctors who do those procedures. For example, regions with a high demand for hip surgeries happen to have lots of hip surgeons, while the patients in those regions may have no more hip disease than others do elsewhere.

There is also a lack of communication. It is good to have someone treating your heart who knows a lot about it. But when a patient has six different specialists, each one treating his or her own specialty without communicating with the other five, this presents a problem. Each specialist sees only one part of the patient's problem, and that specialist may prescribe drugs, recommend surgeries and procedures, and come to conclusions about a person's entire future while looking only at that one part. It is not unusual for a patient to see a neurologist for headache drugs and injections, a rehabilitation doctor for shoulder-pain injections, and a spine surgeon for neck-pain surgery. Each of these doctors may consider different options for treatment without recognizing that all these pains may be connected, and that dividing the patient's treatment into little bits and pursuing one bit of treatment without taking the patient's other parts into account is not the best course. It is crucial to remember that all these problems exist and interact inside the same person's body. They may all be interrelated problems.

Other pressures too, aside from the Flexner report, have encouraged the expansion of the allopathic system. During the mid-twentieth century, the financial giant called the pharmaceutical industry was born. That industry's genesis was closely tied to the chemical industry, and some of America's first drugs were created from chemical dyes, coal tar, and even leftover airplane fuels developed during World War II. These drugs were created to target problems — for example, antibiotics were developed to target organisms that cause infections. Soon, medications were looked at as necessary weaponry in the battle against disease. Doctors were gunslingers, and drugs, their guns. Of course, the gunslinger approach only works if the doctor has clear and specific targets. It works best if the patient is a collection of parts and not an entire, complex person.

In *Anatomy of an Epidemic* (2010), Robert Whitaker outlines how this gunslinger approach began to be used for psychiatric disorders. These disorders, however, were not clear targets. Patients had symptoms and behaviors of schizophrenia, depression, and anxiety, but no diseases had been established. The drugs curbed patients' behaviors and symptoms, but no consideration was given to how these drugs affected the human body and brain. These types of drugs are still used today and produce troublesome results. Sadly, people with these conditions do better in undeveloped countries than they do with modern medicine. This is the damning message of Whitaker's book, and the principle may hold for more than just psychiatric drugs.

For decades, I have personally noticed the growing pressure applied by the pharmaceutical industry — the drug companies. The first thing I noticed was advertising. I hate advertising. They started out by having glossy ads in the medical journals, where they seemed to be the journals' only sponsors. Then, drug companies were taking doctors to lunches, giving them gifts, and offering them high fees to speak at dinners given for their colleagues.

Each new drug enjoys a period of time when its developer has exclusive rights to produce it. After a few years, the patent expires and other companies can use the same chemical formula to make generic versions of that drug. The generics are usually cheaper. Over the years, I saw a rapidly growing number of new drugs, many of which did the same things as the old ones. It seemed like a full-time job to remember all the names and dosages. My colleagues seemed to be doing it, so I felt pressured to keep up with the latest changes. Around this time, I also noticed more visits from drug reps — the paid and mostly commissioned sales force of the pharmaceutical industry. They presented themselves as educators, here to inform doctors about the latest research. The sales aspect of their jobs was largely hidden from sight. They fed me interpretations of statistics on neat little one-page summaries of research papers. They left samples for me to start patients on. Some of the time, they even left me prewritten prescriptions to make it easy for me to prescribe the more expensive new drug rather than the older, cheaper, but equally effective one that I had been using for years. In addition, these reps were not allowed to tell me about circumstances in which the drug could be used "off label" — that is, in a way not specifically listed in its instructions — but they would tell me that other doctors were doing it all the time. In this way, a sales force with no medical background was trying to influence the prescribing practices of trained physicians.

As time went on, studies began to show that these marketing practices were greatly influencing doctors' prescribing habits. Eventually, government regulators imposed limits on the gifts and perks that drug companies could offer. The drug companies have since shifted their strategies, but they still influence the market through offers of paid employment on advisory panels and through third-party market research firms.

Drug companies have become big business and are driven by all the pressures that spur big businesses to put profits above people. The pharmaceutical industry supports the compartmentalized, allopathic approach to health care because it is a profitable one. But the drug companies' interests are not necessarily the patients', and we are seeing more and more how ineffective the allopathic approach can be.

Cholesterol-lowering drugs called statins were developed to treat a small group of people whose cholesterol is so high they are prone to heart attacks at a very early age. But drug companies are not targeting only this small group of people. Instead, they are also marketing statins to normal people who have "above-normal" cholesterol. Now we see statins all over the medical world. Statins are even being recommended for some children! A doctor in the United Kingdom recently suggested they should be offered with fast-food combos — a burger, fries, and a statin.[5] He was joking. I hope.

Studies show us that statins are good at lowering a patient's cholesterol, but what evidence do we have that statins are good for patients in general? The answer is scary: there isn't any. The research studies on statins asked only specific questions about cholesterol levels. Do they reduce hardening of the arteries? Are there fewer signs of inflammation in the blood? Is the cholesterol level lower? Do people have fewer cardiac events over a short period of time? The answers to these questions suggest the drug is good for the drug's intended user — people with cholesterol that is above "normal." But if we ask different, more general questions, we may get a very different answer. For example: do people taking statins live longer, fuller lives with greater overall health? We don't know. The studies of statins aren't asking the questions that are important to the patients and, therefore, aren't getting the answers that are important to the patients.

Sometimes we don't ask the right questions regarding pain treatment, either. A nonprofit organization called the Joint Commission, which accredits hospitals with the aim of improving hospital standards and outcomes, has established standards on pain treatment. These require that every patient be asked about pain, and that any pain complaint be addressed during the medical visit. Usually the simplest way to quickly address a pain complaint is with drugs. The question not asked is: "Is the patient better able to proceed with her life after her pain is addressed?" If she had acute pain, usually she is. If she had chronic pain, maybe she isn't.

In looking for more information we must be wary of what A. W. Kimball defined as statistical "errors of the third kind" — giving the right answer to the wrong question.[6] We have in the past received some definitive answers to the wrong questions. The important questions about chronic pain are enormously complex, and the answers may be uncertain. But if we can tolerate the uncertainty, it may ultimately lead to more helpful information.

Randomized control trials are considered the gold standard of research evidence. But these studies try to reduce the complexity of the questions they ask. And ultimately they give us definitive answers to the wrong questions. These trials normally have many inclusion and exclusion criteria — specific characteristics of the patients or their illness that either allow them to be in the study or keep them from being in the study. These criteria are designed to make the groups more similar and less complicated. The problem is that patients who walk into my office are really complicated and usually don't resemble the patients in the studies at all. So randomized control trials end up telling us little about real-life situations. Information about real-life patients is more complicated to get. It involves tracking our patients' progress and recording tons of information about the details of their lives as they experience various treatments. These are called outcome studies, and they are becoming increasingly more respected. They have a better chance of answering the right questions.

Our approach to pain care costs over half a trillion dollars each year. Despite this, millions of sufferers are disabled by pain, and their number is still growing. If we had the right answers, wouldn't the number be going down? Western scientific progress in the past century is undeniable — the accomplishments include heavier-than-air flying machines and walking on the moon, the discovery of DNA, and the cloning of sheep. But not all steps forward are steps in the right direction, as the statistics of our pain care model suggest.

The baby boomers are aging. They had every expectation that their children would be healthier than their parents were. Their children's generation, however, is now being told that one in three of them will be diabetic. In fact, chronic diseases of many types are growing more common and afflicting sufferers at younger ages. This is shocking.

As a result, we are seeing a grassroots movement toward alternatives. This trend has been chronicled by Harvard University professor David Eisenberg and colleagues, whose 1990 survey on the subject showed that 34 percent of American adults had used at least one unconventional therapy in the previous year, resulting in 425 million office visits. By 1997, 47 percent of Americans had used these therapies within the previous year, making 625 million office visits and incurring an estimated

$30 billion in out-of-pocket expenses.[7] Many of these visits were for pain treatment. Patients are demanding additional low-risk, natural options, which is leading to more research into complementary and alternative medicine — defined as a "group of diverse medical and health care systems, practices, and products that are not generally considered part of conventional medicine."[8] Some conventionally trained doctors have begun collaboration with practitioners of complementary and alternative medicine, leading to a new field of medicine called integrative medicine (IM).

·The Consortium of Academic Heath Centers counts fifty-five of the top university-based medical schools in North America among its members, all of which have some level of commitment to teaching IM in their schools. The National Institutes of Health has established a branch — the National Center for Complementary and Alternative Medicine — devoted to complementary and alternative medicine.

IM focuses on the patient and not the problem. Practitioners of IM spend more time listening to patients' concerns and pay attention to factors affecting the mind, body, and spirit. They recognize that medicine rarely "fixes" what ails the patient. They focus on healing, which allopathic medicine often ignores. Let's not forget, there is a lifelong natural inclination of the body to heal. This health-focused approach affects the questions we ask of our researchers and colleagues, and it changes the conversation with our patients. This has become the way I work as a physician.

Since becoming interested in IM, I have worked to make holistic approaches available to patients. I have spoken on behalf of my patients to their insurers and employers, advocating the coverage of alternative practices. I was successful in getting workers' compensation and motor vehicle accident insurers to cover the costs of alternative therapies. A Canadian clinic I cofounded in the early 1990s was contracted by Canada's national newspaper to diagnose and provide employees with integrative treatment for the growing and costly problem of repetitive strain injuries. In 2006, I was recruited by an insurance company to open a clinic in Tucson, Arizona, offering integrative services to pain patients in the Medicaid system — a group that rarely gets access to such care. But most of these victories seemed small, and the overall attitudes in the field were not changing. Then in 2009, I read a report written by a task force on pain care commissioned by the Office of the Surgeon General of the US Army Medical Department. The report mandated integrative pain care for people in the health care system of the US Departments of Defense and Veterans' Affairs, including their families, which is a significant portion of the pain care system. Big change is coming.

This chapter has discussed how focusing too narrowly on solutions to individuals' problems is not the best approach to pain care. I compare it to fixing a leaky roof by replastering the damaged ceilings in each room. The rooms look better for now, but the next time it rains...

This book is dedicated to changing the conversation on pain care. Let's talk about reshingling the roof instead of replastering the ceilings. Let's talk about your health more than we talk about your problems.

CHAPTER 3

A VISIT WITH AN INTEGRATIVE PHYSICIAN

*The most basic and powerful way to connect to another person
is to listen. Just listen. Perhaps the most important thing
we ever give each other is our attention....A loving silence often has
far more power to heal and to connect than the most well-intentioned words.*

— RACHEL NAOMI REMEN

Meet my patient Janine. Three years ago, she developed a severe pain in her left hip and leg after an injury. The pain now extends all the way down to her ankle. She has had to forgo exercise and is now lamenting all the weight she has been putting on.

Her family doctor was uncomfortable prescribing pain medications and so sent her to a pain clinic. Through the clinic, she tried painkillers, pain-modifying drugs like antiepileptic drugs, numerous antidepressants for pain, and a series of injections.

The painkillers took the edge off, but she was still in pain all the time, and none of the other medications helped. She kept needing higher doses of painkillers because after a few months a lower dose no longer had an effect. Neither her family doctor nor the clinic had anything new to offer, but Janine wanted her life back, so she kept reading and searching. She saw many specialists, surgeons, neurologists, and rehabilitation doctors, but the message was the same: "You'll just have to learn to live with it."

One day, a friend recommended that she make an appointment with a doctor on the other side of town who does things a little differently. That's me. And today is Janine's appointment.

Janine arrives early at my office to check in with my receptionist, who hands her a stack of papers to fill out. Twenty minutes later, Janine's name is called and she is taken into a small room. Soon after, I knock on the door.

"Hi, I'm Heather Tick," I say, extending my hand. I can tell by her tight smile that Janine is nervous, and I smile back, hoping to take the edge off her nervousness.

"I'm glad you're here. Why don't we chat for a bit so that I can get an idea of what's going on with you." I notice that she is dressed nicely and has taken the time to put on makeup. Pain patients often want to appear "normal," to fit in and avoid that feeling of isolation that so often accompanies pain.

"I just have to enter information into the computer as we speak. My apologies for that."

"That's okay," says Janine. "I would have changed into a gown, but there wasn't one."

"You're right. I prefer to talk first. Then you can change and we'll do an examination." I look at her and smile. For the first time, Janine leans back into her chair and seems to relax a bit.

I then ask her to tell me her story. Why she is here. I also need the details about her pain. When it started. How it progressed. Where it is now. After ten minutes, I ask her to clarify some of the information. She apologizes for wandering through the details in an unorganized manner.

"Not to worry," I say. "It's hard to remember what happened when. You have been telling me how your pain affects your life and what important things you want to get back into your life. What we're trying to do is put together the puzzle of your symptoms and pain. We need to figure out as much as we can about it so that I can find the best way to help you get what you want. What you're doing now is laying out all the pieces. So it doesn't matter what order they're in." Janine smiles at this.

I ask her about her diet, not in general, but specific details. How many servings of fruits and vegetables does she eat every day? Does she drink soda? How much coffee, tea, and alcohol does she drink? What kinds of starches does she eat, and exactly what breads and cereals does she use? What does she have for snacks? How much sugar? How much protein and what kinds?

We then discuss her exercise, work, sleep, and stress. Janine willingly provides a pretty complete picture of her lifestyle. I learn about her work and family life, how she feels emotionally, and what her spiritual practices are. After thirty-five minutes, I have come to know quite a bit about this thirty-eight-year-old woman in front of me. Her sense of humor has emerged, and I find her to be bright and sensitive. We are building a friendly patient-doctor relationship. If we are to work together to solve the mystery of her pain and design a therapy to resolve it, we need to work as a team. I have the training and experience that can help diagnose the problem and direct the course of healing; Janine has the power within to follow that course and tap into her body's innate healing power.

I conclude our chat with short questions about past medical problems, family history, and any ongoing medical issues.

"Now you can change into a gown," I say, handing her one. I leave the room for a few minutes to give her privacy.

When I return, I ask Janine to walk back and forth across the room.

"Now walk on your heels." She does. "And now your toes." She does this also. "Now do a squat. Now stand up and raise your arms above your head."

She laughs. "Seriously?" she says. "For a bad hip? No one has ever asked me to do this."

"We're doing a full head-to-toe musculoskeletal exam. The body doesn't know we look at it in parts. You never know where you might find clues."

When the exam is complete, I tell her to dress and that we'll talk some more. While I'm out of the exam room I look over her previous tests, blood work, X-rays, ultrasound results, and an MRI that shows a small herniated disc. When I return, I tell Janine that I think most of her problems are myofascial, which means the pain comes from the muscles and the connective tissues around the muscles, called fascia. Her test results are pretty normal, because X-rays and MRIs don't see the details of the myofascial system. Painkillers and antidepressants do not help these injuries. So I can understand why Janine has been so frustrated. For the next quarter of an hour, I ask her about her goals. What would she like to see happen as a result of this meeting?

"What I would really like," she says, "is to know why I have this excruciating pain in my hip and leg. Why can't anyone tell me that?" I hear frustration in her voice. "I want to get off these narcotic painkillers because they constipate me, and I don't think as well, and I'm pretty much still in pain. And I would like to exercise like I have in the past."

I lean forward in my chair, my hands in my lap. "Okay, those are all reasonable goals." I see the hint of surprise flash across Janine's face. "First of all, let me say I believe that you can get better. There are therapies you haven't tried yet, which could offer improvement." I then talk for a few minutes about the body's natural healing capacity and tell her that, as a doctor, I see my first job as guiding Janine through the process of tapping into that innate power.

"So now let's draw up a list of possible changes that you can make in your lifestyle that will help relieve your pain."

"We can do this now?" says Janine. "Before you do any more tests?"

"Yes, definitely. You can start to make changes tomorrow, if you want."

Janine sits up straight in the chair. "Yes! Let's do it." She gives me the biggest smile I've seen from her yet.

I suggest that she eat protein with every meal, and that she decrease her diet soda from three per day to one. Eventually, she'll want to eliminate soda altogether, but going cold turkey can be hard. Better to take small steps. I explain that our body chemistry changes every time we eat, and that food increases and decreases our inflammation. Janine looks dumbstruck.

"I know that inflammation causes more pain and keeps things from healing," she says, "but I had no idea that my choices make that big of a difference."

I encourage her to find a gentle physical activity that she can do, such as yoga, qi gong, water exercises, or perhaps just walking. Maybe before the next appointment, she could try some of these and see what feels most comfortable to her physically, and also what fits into her schedule and finances.

Finally, I write out an order for blood tests and hand it to her. I also give her a printout of information about diet that has been customized to our discussion. It even includes a recipe for lentil salad.

"This is a first. I am going home with a recipe and not a prescription for another drug! I feel as though you are interested in taking care of all of me, " Janine says. "And you haven't told me I just have to learn to live with it."

As she is leaving, I say to her, "I think you're going to start feeling better sooner than later."

"I can't remember the last time I've felt so hopeful," says Janine. "I'm even excited to give up my diet soda." She laughs and leaves the office, a much more relaxed and happy person than when she arrived.

I tell all of my patients, including Janine: "No one has the right to take away your hope. There are ways to take charge of your health and improve it. It is important to focus on the positive aspects of your health and work at increasing those."

Let's look at how this integrative medicine appointment changed the conversation on Janine's pain care. Some of the components are similar to any doctor visit and some differ.

I knew that Janine would be nervous during our first visit, and so I worked hard to help her relax. It is difficult to be a pain patient and see a new doctor. You never know how the interview will go. Studies show that 50 percent of pain patients who are seeing a new doctor feel that this doctor does not understand what is important to them. As we saw in chapter 2, the focus of an appointment for a doctor is usually finding the diagnosis that is required for the insurance chart. Often, the diagnosis is the end of the conversation. Janine was obviously used to this regular sort of appointment; she was surprised that I wanted to talk to her for a while before she put on a gown. I too need to come up with a diagnosis that will represent this patient on paper; but for IM doctors the diagnosis is only the starting point of the conversation, and we try as much as possible to understand the unique features of each patient. It generally takes longer to get all that information, so both the appointment and the length of time the patient is allowed to speak are longer. All that time costs the system more in the short run, but in the long run, if we can keep patients from getting unnecessary procedures, surgeries, and drugs, this approach potentially will save the system a lot of money and save patients a lot of suffering.

A diagnosis is just a name that we doctors agreed to use for a group of signs and symptoms. Diagnoses can sometimes be useful, because they streamline our thinking and expectations. But sometimes they are not helpful for the same reasons; a person's medical problems are more individual than a diagnosis suggests.[1]

I started with Janine's diagnosis, but I didn't let it limit our conversation. According to this diagnosis, she has a small herniated disc at the point on her spine designated as L4-5, which showed up on an MRI, but from talking to Janine I know her problem is more complicated than that diagnosis suggests. In fact, I anticipate that only a small part of her pain problem is actually a direct result of the disc.[2] She also has some osteo-arthritis, improper posture, myofascial pain, a poor diet, some vitamin deficiencies, a lack of exercise, and too much stress in her life that she isn't acknowledging. Looking at her pain problem this way, I see many more possible causes and many more possible solutions.

The IM process begins with the allopathic medical basics and then goes further. I did a conventional physical examination on Janine and ordered all the appropriate tests, but I also widened the menu a little to include a more complete physical examination than is customary with a pain visit. I look at the whole body for clues to the problem, instead of at only the part that hurts. It surprised Janine when I told her that her head is tilted to the side and she has very tight muscles around her right shoul-der. There is a sore spot in the middle of her back she did not even know about. If I had focused only on the back problem that was the reason for her visit, I would have missed these problems; and if I don't include solu-tions for the neck and shoulder, the back will actually be harder to treat. We will discuss that later on. Instead of seeing myself as the "gunslinger" I described in chapter 2, I see myself as a detective looking for clues to help solve Janine's problems.

In the first interview, I reviewed Janine's diet and explained to her some of the things she could do for herself that can make a difference. "You change your body chemistry every time you eat" is a sentence I find myself repeating often — few people realize how important diet is. I negotiate with patients about what they are willing to change. First they help me understand their habits and priorities, and then they commit to some change. For some patients, these changes start small — as small as eating one vegetable every day. Others are ready to dive in deep and change their habits drastically. It is never one-size-fits-all. In Janine's case, she drinks diet soda daily, eats sweets for energy, and does not have enough healthy proteins and oils in her diet. We discussed how to gradu-ally make changes, and I gave her a handout to remind her about our conversation on diet. We will revise that handout when she is ready for new steps on her journey to a healthier life. We also discussed ways to increase Janine's activity level, which should make her feel better physically and psychologically. Other lifestyle issues will be discussed at the next appointment, because we ran out of time. The focus of the appointment was her health and what she can do to improve it. She has the power to do these things; I am just her coach.

Stress is a factor for all of us. We live in stressful times. For pain patients, there is the added stress of coping with pain at the same time. We cannot separate out what aspects of a person's life are caused by stress or are causing stress. Life is all one big stew...Stress needs to be addressed with Janine, and I will get into that during later appointments.

"You have to learn to live with it" is a sentence pain patients hate to hear. I will discuss with Janine how to balance her acceptance of her current state of health with the hopeful attitude that making healthy changes in her lifestyle can improve her health over time. It is in fact a helpful part of recovery to learn coping skills and learn to live with our pain instead of fighting it, because only rarely is there a pain pill, a surgery, or a procedure that will totally erase chronic pain. So we do have to learn to manage and live with all of our health conditions. But a problem arises when that statement is interpreted to mean there is no hope. Currently it is popular in medicine to say that "chronic pain is a chronic disease." Unfortunately, patients usually interpret this to mean that the condition, like most other chronic diseases, is bound to get worse over time. This is true some of the time — and in some ways chronic pain does resemble a chronic disease.

For example, certain changes take place in the nervous and immune systems, and these changes can perpetuate pain by causing chronic pain patients to be more sensitive to slightly painful or even nonpainful stimuli. A system in our brain and spinal cord is designed to dampen our experience of nonthreatening pain, and chronic pain sometimes causes this system to stop working. A change such as this is an example of neuroplasticity — one of the ways that the brain and nervous system can change themselves. Such changes are used as proof that the pain has changed into a chronic condition. But calling chronic pain a chronic disease assumes that these changes are permanent and that they sentence a person to a lifelong, deteriorating disease state. In fact, these changes can be modifiable, and even reversible, because of neuroplasticity — the same tendency of the brain to change itself. We are at the beginning of understanding how the brain can do this. And some exciting research shows that we can use neuroplasticity to heal ourselves.

I have found that a focus on health is the best way to move the conversation about pain in a positive direction. Most people have never been told that there are things they can do for themselves every day to affect their health and their pain. I join my patients on their journey as a guide. This is how I change the conversation.

Assessing Your Lifestyle

So now it's your turn.

The first step toward managing your pain is to come up with a game plan. And the first step in creating that plan is to determine where you are right now. It's kind of like going to the gym and working with a personal trainer. You don't start with two hundred crunches. You start with a number based on your level of fitness, and as your fitness level increases, so does the number of crunches.

The questions below will help you know where you stand at this moment. Then you can determine what changes you can make in your life that will start you on a path toward healing, health, and less pain.

No one is going to see your answers, so be honest. In fact, there are no right or wrong answers. This information will give you insight into your lifestyle and your habits. You might find areas that need tweaking and areas that are in good shape. Just remember: don't judge yourself. You're doing the best you can right now. Our goal is to make your health and your life — and all that goes with them — the very best they can be.

PERSONAL HEALTH ASSESSMENT

1. Diet

How many servings of the following do you eat each day? Note: a serving is one-half cup or a handful, or in the case of a fruit such as an apple or banana, it is the whole fruit.

Vegetables (raw, cooked, pickled, and so on)

Fruits

Whole grains: quinoa, buckwheat, brown rice (or basmati white rice), whole-grain bread, steel-cut or large-flake rolled oats, and so on[3]

Refined or high-glycemic starches: regular bread, white rice, boxed cereals, white pasta, white potatoes

Proteins: red meat, poultry, fish, eggs

Beans and other legumes plus pulses, such as lentils

Dairy products: milk, cheese, and yogurt, whether made of cow's or goat's milk

Nuts and seeds

Beverages: water, tea, coffee, soda, milk, alcohol, or milk substitutes like coconut, rice, soy, or nut milks

Sweets

Commercial snack foods

How many times a week do you eat in restaurants?

How many times a week do you cook at home?

How many times a week do you use commercially prepared, processed foods at home?

How often do you get drowsy after you eat?

Do you ever get jittery after you eat?

Do you have cravings for starches and sugary foods? Salty foods?

How often do you have bowel movements? Are they soft and easy to pass?

2. Exercise

How often do you exercise?

How long do you spend exercising?

How active are you in your normal daily activities?

What are the types of activities you do for exercise? List how often and how long you spend with each activity.

Do you enjoy exercise?

Is there a particular physical activity that you enjoy?

3. Breathing

Do you smoke? If so, how often?

When you are concentrating on an activity, do you ever notice that you are holding your breath?

When you are nervous or stressed, do you ever notice that you are holding your breath?

Do you know any specific breathing exercises?

Do you practice them regularly?

4. Sleep

How many hours do you sleep each night?

How often do you wake up during that time?

Do you wake up refreshed?

Do you feel drowsy during the day?

Are there computers or electronics in your bedroom?

Do you use the computer or watch television during the hour before you go to sleep?

Is your bedroom totally dark at night without a crack of light or lights from electronic devices? (Red light is acceptable.)

Do you have difficulty falling asleep? If so, describe.

Do you have difficulty getting back to sleep if you wake up in the night? If so, describe.

5. Home Environment

Do you have any concerns about toxic exposure in your home, such as heavy metals in old paint, in water pipes, from smokers, or from pesticide used in the past?

Do you regularly use pesticides inside your home?

Do you use pesticides outside of your home?

Do you use chemical cleaners, or natural cleaners such as vinegar, baking soda, borax, and lemon?

Continued on next page

5. Home Environment (continued)

Do you use plastic containers for food storage?

Do you microwave your food in plastic?

Do you filter your water for drinking? For bathing?

6. Work Environment

Are you comfortable in your workstation at your place of work?

Do you know if there are any adjustable elements to your workstation? If there are, have you adjusted them so that you are comfortable?

Does your employer have a professional who can help you make your workstation more user-friendly?

Do you experience discomfort during your workday or after your workday? If so, is it relieved by the next day?

Do you have discomfort that gets worse as the week progresses?

7. Stress

Do you feel stressed? What does this mean to you?

Do you feel joy at least once a day?

Do you feel gratitude at least once a day?

Do you feel anxious? How much of the time?

  When you wake up in the morning?

  When you wake up in the night?

  When you have a quiet time?

  All day long?

Can you share these feelings with someone important in your life?

Do the important people in your life know your emotions?

Do you feel there are people in your life who fully accept you and still love you in spite of any "bad" emotions like anger or fear?

Is it hard to say "I love you"?

Is it hard to say "I am angry with you"?

Is it harder to say "I love you" or "I am angry with you"?

Do you fly off the handle and get angry?

Is anyone in your home physically violent?

Are you ever physically violent?

8. Spiritual Practices

Do you have a religious or spiritual connection?

How important is that to you?

Do you share that part of your life with others?

Is gratitude a part of your religious or spiritual awareness?

According to an ancient saying, "everywhere you go, there you are." Your habits and patterns stay with you. If changes must happen, we need a starting point. In the coming chapters we will discuss how to change some of your habits and improve your ability to heal.

PART II

PAIN SOLUTIONS

CHAPTER 4

THE HEALING DIET
Lost Food Traditions

Eat food. Not too much.
Mostly plants.

— MICHAEL POLLAN,
In Defense of Food: An Eater's Manifesto

Before societies existed, we humans occupied most of our time with food. We spent our days foraging and hunting for it, preparing it, and eating it. Eventually, we learned to sow and harvest it, which allowed us to live and work in communities. Then the Industrial Revolution led to agricultural advancements and cheap, high-calorie foods that required little preparation. These new foods would make meals convenient for the growing blue-collar workforce in urban centers. Since the start of the Industrial Revolution, we have drifted farther and farther from our original diets, toward more convenient ones — diets of cheaper calories that require less preparation time. Our eating habits have changed too. While our ancestors would spend hours eating and savoring their food, we see no problem with eating our lunches on the go — sitting on a bus or, worse, while running to catch one. Although our new food customs make eating easier, they are not necessarily better. Cheap calories do not mean nutritious ones, and fast food does not mean healthy food. But just how bad for us are these processed, empty calories? How much does our new food affect our health?

At the turn of the twentieth century, Weston Price, a dentist, traveled through regions of the world occupied by indigenous cultures that had not yet been affected by trade with industrialized nations. He was interested in the eating customs and diets of indigenous groups living in remote regions of Ireland, Switzerland, Polynesia, South America, and the Arctic. He found that the diets of these groups varied greatly from region to region, depending on what foods were naturally abundant. Some diets were vegetarian or vegan, while others were based on dairy products or fish or other animals. All groups ate lots of fermented foods and had different diets for special situations — for example, expectant mothers ate a diet different from that of the rest of the population. In addition, he observed that none of the groups refined their foods, and of course, he found no refined flour or sugar whatsoever. Although the diets of many groups were high in fats, even saturated fats and cholesterol, Price found that those groups showed no signs of the chronic diseases that were beginning to plague the developed world. He found no evidence of dental cavities, ear infections, tuberculosis, heart disease, or the need for orthodontics. All of the indigenous groups Price investigated considered food to be sacred, and they treated it with respect.

Twenty years after his first trip, Price returned to those same regions. On his second trip, he made a devastating discovery: all of the indigenous groups that had begun to trade with the developed world also developed the diseases of the developed world. The more flour and sugar the indigenous groups ate, the more they suffered from dental diseases, chronic illness, and infections. As their traditional eating patterns changed, their health deteriorated drastically.[1]

Most North Americans are overfed but undernourished.[2] Our new

foods and eating habits have caused an epidemic of diet-related illnesses — diabetes, arthritis, and cardiovascular disease, among others.
Chronic pain is often a natural consequence of
these illnesses and of poor nutrition in general.
What you eat affects how you feel. When we do
not get the nutrients we need, our cells cannot
heal. When we eat the wrong types of foods, we
increase the inflammation in our body, which
can cause pain. If we overeat empty calories, we
gain weight and put more strain on our joints,
ligaments, and tendons. This adds to our pain
on a macrolevel: it causes more wear and tear on
our spine and joints. It also adds to our pain on a
microlevel: it increases inflammation.

Some of the developed Western countries
— France is a good example — maintain strong
traditional eating patterns and are faring better
than America in overall health. Unfortunately,
much of the rest of the world aspires to eat like
Americans. They want what we have: abundance
and indulgence. They want, for example, a wide
array of what should be seasonal foods to be
available all year long. They want fast foods, full
of chemicals and preservatives, just like we have.
This will continue to be a growing international
problem until there is widespread recognition
of the impact of nutrition on health — until we
return to the traditional patterns of food production and preparation.

> Proper diet helps control weight. Carrying too much weight aggravates pain in the back, knee, foot, and hip and can promote abnormal posture, causing neck pain. By one estimate, there is a four-pound reduction in stress on the knee joint for every pound lost by an overweight individual. Even a modest weight loss may significantly lighten the load on your joints.
>
> "The accumulated reduction in knee load for a 1-pound loss in weight would be more than 4,800 pounds per mile walked," writes Stephen P. Messier of Wake Forest University in Winston-Salem, North Carolina.[3]

The Food Industry

Before the advent of the food industry, food business was conducted at
a marketplace (usually outdoors), where individuals could buy products

grown or created by other members of the community. Food business now entails a huge industry supporting multiple big businesses, which include corporate farmers, processing plants, the chemical industry, the pharmaceutical industry, lobbyists, advertisers, and the industries supported by advertisements, such as television and magazines.[4] To be healthy, we in North America need to change our eating habits. Unfortunately, these habits are difficult to change because big business is directly dependent on them, and the food industry is doing everything it can to stifle this change.

Like the tobacco industry, the food industry uses marketing to maintain and establish new traditions. In 2009, the fast-food industry alone spent $4.2 billion on advertising, which convinced us to spend $110 billion on their products.[5] Like the tobacco manufacturers, the food industry hires scientists to make their products more addictive — to produce foods we can't stop ourselves from eating. They do not disclose all of what is in manufactured foods, but these foods include fat, sugar, salt, and worse — stabilizers, pesticides, antibiotics, preservatives, and pink, foamy, texture modifier.

SAD

The acronym for the "standard American diet" is SAD...and it is.

The sugar that they add to their products, along with refined flour and other starches, spikes our blood sugar and then causes it to drop, leaving us cranky, tired, and craving more food. Over several decades, these new traditions have encouraged us to overeat. *The Agriculture Fact Book*, produced by the Department of Agriculture, estimates that between 1970 and 2000, the average American's calorie intake went up by 530 calories per day.[6] Three thousand extra calories gains you one pound of weight, which means these extra calories would cause an individual to gain one pound every week — fifty-two pounds a year. Is it any wonder that obesity and diabetes are epidemic?

Our bodies have natural instincts that are supposed to guide us toward the nutritional balance that keeps us healthy. Somehow, our brain and body know what we need and have a natural tendency to seek it out.

Our bodies are looking for nutrition, and if the food we eat has none, then we keep eating. At the same time, the body knows when it has had enough. If you are hungry and all you have is a table full of bananas, you will eat a banana. If you are still hungry, you may eat a second, but you are unlikely to go right on to a third and fourth unless you are really starving. You will have had enough bananas. But what about those chocolate cream-filled cookies, that gigantic bag of chips, or the extralarge portion of something greasy and full of chemicals from that fast-food joint down the road? We don't have a natural shutoff switch for those products, because our bodies developed before we invented processed foods. The food industry makes fortunes off of foods we cannot stop ourselves from eating.

A typical grocery store in the United States or Canada has about fifty thousand different items in its food aisles. Very few of those items, however, should be called food. Most of the mixes, sauces, juices, and canned foods are full of chemical stabilizers and preservatives and have no nutritional value. The fluffy white breads and pastries, and most of the commercially prepared cereals, contain as much nutrition as a spoonful of table sugar, and they will raise your blood sugar faster. I've heard it joked that the cardboard boxes in grocery stores may be more nutritious than some of the food products themselves — at least the boxes have some fiber. I start my nutrition lectures with this advice: "If it wasn't food one hundred years ago, it probably isn't food today." If you make most of your food choices with that in mind, you will heal your body and prevent diseases. In addition, you will improve our planet by curbing pollution and contributing to healthy farming practices.

Allopathic Nutrition

After the Flexner report and the closing of alternative medical schools, medical education in the United States shifted its focus from healing to pharmacology. Although many patients think that medical doctors are a good source for nutritional information, most North American doctors have received only a few hours of education on nutrition. There are doctors who have an interest and expertise in nutrition, but this usually means they have trained themselves outside of their allopathic medical education. Most of our medical schools base their nutrition curriculum on the food pyramid, which encourages the consumption of grains without specifying that they must be whole grains and minimally processed.[7] Most of the conventionally trained dietitians have been taught this same curriculum and are restricted in what they are allowed to recommend. This curriculum has more to do with politics than with science; the food industry lobbies our government to subsidize farmers who grow millions of hectares of only a handful of different grain crops, and big business is interested in promoting those crops as an essential component of our diet.[8] Remarkably, while grain-based, low-fat diets have been promoted since the 1960s, they have never been based on research. As it turns out, these diets cause heart disease, diabetes, and obesity. It has taken mavericks in the health field to push back against conventional curriculums and do proper research. This new research is just now filtering through the official channels of government agencies and professional health organizations. Until now, people have been largely left to inform themselves on proper nutrition.

I was taught the same nutritional curriculum as other allopathic doctors. I, however, was also raised by parents who were immigrants to Canada and who held old-fashioned food values. Growing up, we always cooked meals at home from fresh ingredients. We did eat grains, mostly bread and cooked whole-grain cereals, but packaged and processed foods were a rarity at our house. We ate tons of salad, fruit, and cooked (I must say, usually overcooked) vegetables that were in season. My mother always preferred to know exactly where our food came from. I remember there was a farm family that used to come to our neighborhood and sell farm-fresh eggs. I was always excited to bring out a big bowl for them to count the eggs into. It felt so special to have eggs brought to us by the farmers who raised the chickens. My mother distrusted mixes and processed foods because she suspected that they were full of chemicals.

It turns out she was right, even though in those days the labels did not disclose ingredients. Restaurants were an occasional treat and never a regular event. My sister and I both learned to cook at a young age, and when we had families of our own, we cooked most of our families' meals as well. I learned many good lessons at a young age that gave me a life-long interest in healthy food. I received a better nutrition education at home than I did at medical school.

Nutrition and Chemistry

Sometimes when I suggest to a colleague that dietary changes could help a patient, I am met with skepticism. Some doctors feel that the dietary solution is too complicated, that the patient won't follow the recommendations, or that nutritional medicine is unproven and may cause harm. Most of these doctors, however, would not hesitate to prescribe a drug. They want to see the same kind of research that is done on drugs done on diets and nutrition. They act as though the side effects of food and supplements are similar to, or even riskier than, those of drugs. There is a lot of nutrition research out there, but the best nutrition research does not look like drug research — it isn't always double-blind and placebo controlled. This is because, to be meaningful, nutrition research must study the effect of a whole diet on a whole body's chemical makeup, and not just the effect of a single nutrient on a single organ as though it were a drug, like a statin.

You will see in chapter 7 that I do encourage the use of some supplements. But the basis for a healthy body chemistry is a diet of a variety of whole, unprocessed foods rather than pills. For the most part, we cannot treat individual nutritional components as though they were drugs. For example, when it was shown that those who ate carrots had less breast cancer, and that those who ate broccoli had less bowel cancer, some scientific gunslingers got together and came up with an extract — beta-carotene — and thought of it as a magic bullet for cancer prevention. When tested, however, beta-carotene proved disappointing. This is because the extract is not enough. A whole host of carotenoids, combined with fiber and other nutrients, supply the health protection of carrot-ness and broccoli-ness.

Inflammation and Food

The chemical makeup of your body is like the soil that we grow plants in. For your body to grow and heal, your chemical makeup needs to be full of balanced nutrients — just as soil has to be full of balanced nutrients for us to raise beautiful and healthy plants. This simple principle has not been incorporated into the conventional medical understanding about health and healing. Nutrition research has shown that we can change the chemistry of our bodies to improve metabolism and encourage healing throughout our lives. In fact, every time you eat — every day, at every meal — you change your body's internal chemistry, for better or for worse. Food promotes healing or does just the opposite.

Food is especially helpful in balancing inflammation. Inflammation is the reaction of our body to substances that may harm us, such as bacteria, viruses, and damaged cells. Since ancient times, inflammation has been described as redness, heat, swelling, and pain. A few simple mechanisms were thought to be responsible for these reactions. In recent years, we have been learning a lot more about the inflammatory response and about its far-reaching effects on our health.

The inflammatory response was initially thought to be the domain of the immune system. We recently discovered, however, that it's actually the result of a complex dance of chemical mediators that have an impact on every cell type and organ system. Inflammatory processes are responsible for most of the damaging effects we see as a result of diseases. These responses are the final common pathway for conditions that include infections, arthritis, diabetes, heart disease, cancer, and muscle pain. But as it turns out, inflammation is involved in healing us too. It is precisely because both the injury and healing systems overlap that we have to treat inflammation with care. Anti-inflammatory drugs are not the panacea for all illness. Sometimes they are useful and even necessary, but they can have dramatic effects that derail not only the bad side of inflammation but also the healing system. This is where nutrition comes in; foods and nutrients can reduce inflammation and the number of free radicals and leave the healing part of the inflammatory process intact.

Oxidative stress is part of the inflammatory process that involves reactive oxygen species (ROS). ROS are important for understanding the connection between inflammation, disease, and healing.[9] Oxygen is necessary for life, and yet we hear a great deal of confusing information about antioxidants, usually in a context that makes oxygen sound like the enemy. In fact, it is, again, all about balance. Our cells need oxygen to produce energy. It is necessary for life. But under certain circumstances our body produces ROS or other free radicals, which are high-energy particles, kind of like little out-of-control bumper cars zipping around our system and damaging our cells. Some ROS are produced by our body during normal metabolism. Others are stimulated by outside influences, such as the wrong foods (too much sugar, refined foods, fried foods...), smoking, overexposure to the sun, X-rays, and certain chemicals. Nutrition is the most powerful way for us to tip the balance of inflammation toward healing. Antioxidants are molecules, mostly from foods and supplements, that can deactivate the ROS and make them harmless. ROS also play a role in starting out the healing process, because they activate an immune response that encourages our healing forces, such as white blood cells and growth factors. This is why balance is important; ROS are not necessarily bad, but we need antioxidants available to neutralize them if they get out of hand.

INFLAMMATION = PAIN

When I tell my pain patients there is a way for them to reduce the inflammation in their bodies, they immediately make the connection between increased inflammation and pain and realize I am giving them a way to lessen their pain.

Diet is more powerful in preventing the common diseases than either drugs or medical care.[10] It has been known throughout the ages that foods are important for healing and optimal health. In primitive societies, there were traditional foods for certain life events such as childbearing and old age. There were herbs and roots to be ingested or mixed into topical preparations and used as remedies. Indeed, there were medicinals from herb gardens before modern chemicals were ever invented. A search of the botanical literature on functional foods — foods that can have a beneficial effect on the internal processes of our cells — turns up many pages of references from all countries and prominent institutions. There is strong science behind the idea that food promotes health, and we need to make use of it. When we are talking about an intervention as thoroughly time tested and safe as eating properly, we do not have to wait for "safety data," as we would with drugs. You can improve your body chemistry today by making good food choices.

We Are What We Eat, Digest, and Absorb

The information that follows is useful for anybody in pain. I am not a gastroenterologist or stomach specialist, however; so if you have any stomach conditions, you should see a health care provider. Bowel symptoms such as the ones discussed here can be the early signs of serious diseases like cancer and inflammatory diseases. You should not self-diagnose or self-treat. If your doctors tell you there is nothing seriously wrong with the structures of your digestive tract, then you can use the information that follows to improve your digestion, reduce your pain, and enhance your overall health.

Our gut is a gateway between the outside and inside worlds. The gut, or digestive tract, is a continuous tube that extends from the mouth, through the esophagus, the stomach, the small and large intestine, and the rectum, to the anus. What is inside the tract is actually considered to be still outside the body; something must pass through the wall of the tube to become part of our body fluids and cells. The tract wall is a membrane called the mucosa. A healthy mucosa is a barrier to foreign materials, which are allowed into the body only after they have been well processed, or digested. Sometimes, an unhealthy mucosa allows undigested, inappropriate particles into the body. This is a serious condition called leaky gut. The gut behaves like a sieve, allowing toxic molecules into the body.

Eighty percent of the immune system lies inside the body, just beyond the mucosa, in the gut. In the case of leaky gut, inappropriate particles meet the immune system, which reacts to them as foreign invaders, causing inflammation. If the assault is short-lived, as in an episode of food poisoning, the inflammation settles down over a few days and the integrity of the mucosa is restored. If the assault is continuous, as in the case of free radical damage, food intolerance, true food allergy, or the imbalance of normal bacteria, the result is constant low-level inflammation. This type of inflammation affects the entire body.

Leaky gut is commonly caused by an imbalance of microorganisms in the gut. It is best treated with a balanced diet that includes healthy gut bacteria called probiotics. Prebiotics — nutrients that help feed probiotics — are also important. Probiotics are found in yogurt and fermented foods. To avoid leaky gut, avoid excessive sugar and refined carbohydrates, unnecessary antibiotics, foods that contain antibiotics or hormones, and foods that are overexposed to plastics.

WE ARE OUTNUMBERED

The bowel contains more microorganisms – bacteria, yeasts, viruses, and parasites – than the number of human cells that make up our body.[11] These organisms are microbes, and together they are called the microbiome. An extensive study on the microbiome is currently being done at the National Institutes of Health called the Human Microbiome Project. A healthy microbiome keeps the mucosa healthy and helps us digest and absorb our food.

The microbiome affects our immune system, our susceptibility to infection, and our development of IBS, allergies, eczema, asthma, and maybe even obesity.[12] Sometimes certain microbes in our gut reproduce too much or move to the wrong part of the tract. This leads to an unbalanced, unhealthy microbiome, which is called dysbiosis. Dysbiosis is the main cause of leaky gut.

In North America, we have accepted constipation and rising rates of bowel cancer as normal. In a well-known study of bowel function in primitive societies, Dr. Denis Burkitt described people who had three bulky bowel movements per day, one after each meal. They almost never developed bowel cancer.[13] Naturally, things are different in our nonprimitive society. When I take the history of a patient, I always ask about bowel habits. People often tell me they think they have normal bowel habits if they move their bowels every two or three days. And in medical school, I was taught that this frequency of bowel movements was perfectly acceptable. Meanwhile, the National Cancer Institute in the United States reports that, each year, fifty in every one hundred thousand people are likely to get colon or rectal cancer.[14]

Constipation causes many problems. I define normal bowel habits as regular, easy-to-pass bowel movements at least twice a day. When food is digested, we produce free radicals and toxic substances. The longer these substances are left in contact with the lining of the bowel, the more time they have to cause damage. Consequently, infrequent bowel movements can cause bowel disorders, including cancer. Additionally, constipation can cause cramping, painful trapped gas, and the development of diverticula — small outpouchings in the bowel wall that cause pain, bleeding, and infections. There are dietary solutions to all of these problems.

Fiber, especially insoluble fiber, softens stool and speeds up its movement through the bowel. In addition, an insoluble fiber absorbs toxics and minimizes their absorption into the bowel wall. Minerals, especially magnesium and calcium, are also helpful. Adequate magnesium relaxes bowel muscles and relieves bowel pain, establishing normal bowel habits. Lastly, antioxidants help by neutralizing free radicals. Fiber, magnesium, calcium, and antioxidants can be found in vegetables, fruits, seeds, nuts, and whole grains.

Constipation is also associated with two other conditions — irritable bowel syndrome (IBS) and gastroesophageal reflux disease (GERD).[15] Individuals with IBS have bowels that overreact to stressors of all kinds, including specific food groups. The syndrome is often associated with fibromyalgia and chronic pain. Individuals with GERD get heartburn caused by food and acid flowing up the esophagus, instead of down. When dealing with IBS and GERD patients, I encourage them to think of their condition as a complaint from their bowel about their dietary choices. Then I help them modify their diet, which usually solves their bowel problems and improves any other body pain they have as well. Oftentimes, IBS and GERD sufferers react badly to a particular food or group of foods. Keeping a food and symptom diary can help you figure out which foods bother you. Sometimes it will be a specific food or food group, such as gluten or grains, and in other instances it will be a *combination* that is not tolerated. For example, tomatoes may be fine for some people, but not if eaten with onions or coffee. I cover other natural and supplement solutions in chapter 7.

Using medications for IBS is almost always unnecessary. Some of the medications used for IBS have turned out to be dangerous and have even caused deaths. I discuss the drugs used for IBS and GERD in chapter 9.

A Case of Malnutrition

Joe is a forty-eight-year-old lawyer with a successful practice. He eats fast food for breakfast and lunch, and he eats dinners at home several times a week. He drinks three to four cups of coffee every day, at least three cans of diet cola every day, and two to three bottles of beer five nights a week. He is mildly overweight and carries his excess weight around his waist like a spare tire. He does not like vegetables. Joe has reduced his smoking to five cigarettes a day. He often has heartburn, and most days he takes pills for it.

Joe's busy work schedule doesn't let him exercise regularly, but he plays hockey once every week or two and wishes he could play tennis. He has episodes of knee pain and shoulder pain and almost always has neck pain. Occasionally he "puts his back out" and has to take some time off work. At the office, he does a lot of computer work and sits at his desk for most of the day. He has an expensive chair but has never adjusted it.

When he talks on the phone, he often cradles the receiver between his ear and his shoulder while he jots down notes.

The new managing partner at his law firm is someone he has never gotten along with, and this has caused some friction at work. His wife is supportive of his job, but she is busy with her own career and with getting their twenty-two-year-old daughter, Sarah, settled in her new apartment in a town nearby. Sarah has just gotten her first job and calls her mother often for help. Their son has just been accepted into an expensive private business school, and Joe worries about the high tuition fees and the current economy.

The pain in Joe's neck and right shoulder is interfering with his sleep, and this in turn is interfering with his work. His doctor gave him nonsteroidal anti-inflammatories and sleeping pills. He has had steroid shots in his rotator cuff for tendinitis. None of these treatments has helped him.

The first time Joe comes to see me, he's late for the appointment. He rushes in and tells me he's very busy and has to be out of the office by a particular time. He has several important things to do afterward. He also tells me he's going to be traveling a lot over the next two months and cannot come for treatment until he's finished traveling. He is stressed and fidgets while in his chair; he can't find a comfortable position. Joe clearly has a lot of areas I could work on, but I choose the one that will make the biggest difference: his diet.

I ask about the specifics of Joe's diet, and he tells me he understands that he doesn't eat well. He suggests he should return to the healthy eating habits of his youthful, more athletic days. He does not think he will ever be able to give up the pills for heartburn or the cigarettes, but he agrees to begin a series of small changes. He will eat more vegetables every day and get off the subway one stop early so he can do more walking every morning.

Two weeks later, he returns for treatment and to discuss his progress. He has done well with the veggies and has decided on his own to swap his usual bagel for breakfast for a slice of whole wheat toast and eggs. He likes the morning walk and has lengthened it to two subway stops. He reports he has more energy and sleeps better. He is now ready to hear about vitamins and to set a date for reducing the number of cigarettes he smokes.

Joe continues this program for six weeks and has weekly treatment sessions for his tight, sore muscles. He is seeing improvement in his physical condition and starts to really believe that he can heal himself by simply making lifestyle changes. He admits that he lost hope before and thought of himself as an "old man." He recognizes the rut he was in — he felt stressed, did not look after himself, and grew even more stressed as his physical condition deteriorated. He sees this trend reversing and is excited about eating well, losing weight, exercising more, and feeling younger. Exercise is reducing his shoulder pain, which does not wake him up at night anymore, and he no longer needs any painkillers for it. Even his friends and coworkers are commenting that he seems in a better mood and more energetic. His wife is thrilled to have "the man she married" back again.

At my last office visit with Joe, he explains that when he first came to see me everything in his life seemed out of control. Now he feels back in control. I ask what helped him see that he could take charge.

"It was a line you always say about changing your body chemistry every time you eat," he says. "That just stuck with me from then on, and I started making good choices. When I saw how my choices were actually enough to make me feel better, I just kept going and taking charge of more areas of my life."

Your Food Choices

When I first assess a new patient for chronic illness or pain, a diet history is part of the assessment. I see daily proof of the old adage "You are what you eat." I ask people if they eat vegetables and fruit. Almost everyone says yes. Then comes what for many is the harder question: "How many servings of fruit and how many servings of vegetables did you have yesterday?" Far too often, the question is followed by silence as I wait, hoping they are trying to count up large numbers. Then comes the truth: "Well, I don't eat them every day. I had an apple on Tuesday."

So the first order of business is to get people to improve their diets by adding more vegetables and fruits. I explain that eating habits affect pain because diet can either increase inflammation or decrease it. Diet can nourish your cells or leave them vulnerable to further damage.

When dealing with diet, I try to add healthy products before I take away the less healthy ones. I want people to like the process and not feel that I am depriving them of something they are used to eating. A nutritional strategy helps people take charge of their health and lets them see the connection between pain and their overall health. There are times when I prescribe necessary medications, but people are more likely to leave my office with a recipe for lentils or chicken soup than a pharmaceutical prescription.

Veggies and Fruit

The Reagan administration tried to get ketchup declared a vegetable so they could serve french fries and ketchup as part of the school lunch program and count it as two vegetables. Let us be clear: neither french fries nor ketchup should be considered a vegetable. While they may have once been vegetables, processing has destroyed any nutritional value they ever had. You can still eat them once in a while for a treat; just don't count them in your nutrition tally at the end of the day.

I tell my patients that my goal is for them to eat and learn to enjoy ten servings (a serving is about a handful) a day of mostly veggies and some fruits. But I always start slowly and set a goal they think they can achieve. These are some of the toughest negotiations I have ever had — getting people who think they hate veggies to agree to having something green on their plates. If necessary, we aim for just one serving a day to start. We talk specifically about which vegetables. I tell patients that corn and white-flesh potatoes don't count. Sometimes they want to eat the same choice every day — peas, for example. Other times they want more variety.

On subsequent visits, they admit it was not as terrible as they had feared. Then, if they think they are ready, we increase the target number. Over time, I encourage people to experiment with different types of veggies and fruits. We should be eating a rainbow on our plates — green, red, orange, yellow, and purple. There are tons of different veggies and fruits, and I am constantly discovering new ones myself. I discovered kale a few years ago when it was delivered to my home in the weekly basket of organics I had signed up for with a local farm group. And I just picked up collard greens for the first time last month because I read a recipe for them. There is an amazing array of raw-food cookbooks (is that an oxymoron?) that deal only with vegetables.

There is science behind a veggie-and-fruit prescription. Vegetables contain lots of fiber. An example is cellulose, a fiber found in many vegetables. Fiber gives bulk to our bowel movements and catches fat as well as toxic molecules, such as free radicals and pollutants, that we are better off not absorbing into our system. Vegetables and fruits also contain vitamins, minerals, and flavonoids — chemicals that act as antioxidants.

Here are a few of the beneficial components in fruits and vegetables that we have research on:

- Lycopene from tomatoes is a member of the carotenoid family, a group of colorful plant compounds that are potent antioxidants.
- Silymarin, found in artichokes, is another powerful flavonoid with antioxidant activity. Silymarin helps keep liver enzymes active so they can continue their detoxification of harmful substances in the body.
- Indole-3-carbinol is in cruciferous vegetables such as cabbage, brussels sprouts, cauliflower, collards, and broccoli. It helps activate enzymes in the detoxification pathway and helps reduce an imbalance of estrogen by metabolizing estrogens. See chapter 9 for an explanation of the relationship between estrogen and pesticides and plastics.

- Eating berries and pomegranates would be healthy if only because of the joyful riot of color and taste. The bonus is that they contain a variety of flavonoids, flavanols, and quercetin — antioxidants all. The more research that gets done on these precious little fruits, the more we realize how beneficial they are for our health. Organics taste even better. Is there anything as wonderful as the tiny wild blueberries from the forest floor that are blue through and through?

Veggies from the Sea

Few of us in the Western world eat much seaweed. But we should. The earth's farmland has been washed almost clean of iodine, and so the foods we grow have little of this important mineral. Today, we can get good quantities of iodine from fish and seaweed. Natural sea salt doesn't have much iodine, but I would still recommend it over other forms of table salt, which sometimes have iodine added.

Iodine is essential for the function of the thyroid and other organs, and a sluggish thyroid can mean muscle pain and delayed healing.[16] Iodine has also been documented as influencing breast health, and it is likely important for ovarian and prostate health as well.[17]

Carbohydrates and the Glycemic Index

Carbohydrates, or carbs, include breads, grains, cereals, pastas, and more. These days, carbs are getting a bad rap. This is mainly because the market is flooded with refined versions of carbs that consist mostly of wheat with an unnaturally high glycemic index.

The glycemic index (GI) is a measure of how fast a food turns into sugar once you eat it.[18] The scale ranges from o to 100, where 100 describes how fast blood sugar rises when an individual eats straight glucose. Glucose is the sugar molecule our cells use to make energy; it is what is measured in a blood sugar test. Sucrose is table sugar, made of an attached glucose and fructose molecule, and since it requires more time to be broken down than glucose alone, it has a GI of about 62. That means, foods with GIs of about 62 or above turn into sugar in your body faster than sugar does. You might as well eat out of the sugar bowl.

Instant oats have a GI of 65. Some versions of rolled oats are also in the 60s. Steel-cut oats, also called Irish oats, and most rolled oats have a GI closer to 50. The foods with a lower GI are healthier for us, so you generally want to stay below 55.

Most white breads have a GI in the region of 70. The traditional French baguette rates 57, but to achieve this score it needs to be made from a type of wheat available only in France. Some of the commercially prepared cereals have a surprisingly high GI, even the ones promoted for weight loss. When checking a particular food's GI, you will discover that a lot of foods you never suspected are likely to cause a spike in your blood sugar. Get in the habit of checking a book or an online database for the GI of the foods you are eating. This is a good online database: www.glycemicindex.com.

ADVICE FOR BUSY FOLKS

Steel-cut oats take twenty to thirty minutes to cook. Try cooking them the night before and then heating them up with a little water in the morning for a fast, healthy breakfast.

When you eat a food that is high on the glycemic index, your blood sugar spikes and your body quickly compensates by secreting hormones such as insulin to lower it. This usually causes your blood sugar level to drop below the optimal range. This drop usually happens about two hours after you eat, and it makes you feel fatigued, irritable, and hungry for anything that will quickly raise your blood sugar again. That hunger is called "carb cravings," and it puts you on a roller coaster of rising and falling blood sugar levels. Your body chemistry gets into a proinflammatory state, which means more pain. This increases oxidative stress, which causes tissue damage, weight gain, and eventually insulin resistance or prediabetes, which means even more pain.

The fastest way to correct the problem is to eat a low-glycemic diet. This will help solve the metabolic problems, reduce inflammation, and cut out your cravings for the wrong foods. While you are working to curb the carb-craving phase, it often helps to eat five small meals a day with some protein — vegetable or animal protein — in each meal. Once you are no longer craving the foods that spike your blood sugar, you should move to three meals a day with a long fast between dinner and breakfast and five hours between your other meals. Some people will need snacks due to rapid metabolism or extremes in exercise.

Research has shown that low-glycemic meals promote lower insulin and higher circulating levels of the hormone leptin. This balance leads to reduced food consumption, which can help to control obesity and related disorders, including insulin resistance and type 2 diabetes.[19] This is a win-win proposition: you reduce inflammation as well as weight-related pain.[20]

Nonstarch Carbohydrates

There are both good and bad sources of carbs. The ones we think of most readily are starches like bread, pasta, rice, potatoes, and cereals. These are also the ones most likely to spike our blood sugar. Beans and other legumes, lentils, seeds, nuts, and steamed whole grains are also sources of carbohydrates and are high in fiber, vitamins, minerals, and healthy oils. Vegetables also contain carbohydrates, even though we seldom think of them that way.

Protein

As I continue taking the dietary history of a patient, I ask what kinds of proteins they eat. I can approve of almost every category, but I try to encourage patients to choose unprocessed foods, organic if possible. Wild-caught fish from cold waters, grass-fed animals, and free-range poultry and eggs are all excellent protein sources. Research supports eating food that has been naturally raised. It tastes better and has a different nutritional balance. For example, grass-fed beef contains higher levels of omega-3 oils. Omega-3 oils are most commonly found in fish, but good quantities are also found in different animal products if the animals were allowed to roam free to peck or graze in a natural setting. In addition to appreciating the improved nutrition and taste, I find that I eat less food when it is naturally raised or organic. It is as though my body knows when I am eating nutritious food and is satisfied with more quality and less quantity.

North Americans eat too much protein.[21] Most adults can easily satisfy their total protein needs even if they reduce their intake of animal protein to three ounces, three times a week or even eliminate it altogether. If you eat smaller amounts of meat, poultry, eggs, and fish, you can buy better quality. Then, use vegetables, beans, lentils, and whole grains to fill yourself up. It's a healthy way to eat.[22]

Eggs are a source of protein and fats. They also contain a carotenoid called lutein, a yellow pigment that is beneficial for our eyes. If the chickens are free-range, are given quality feed, and are free to peck around in dirt, then the eggs naturally have omega-3 oils. Factory-farmed eggs from chickens — both of which are covered in feces — raised in cramped quarters are more likely to contain salmonella.[23] These chickens are highly stressed, which naturally affects the health of their eggs. I like to buy eggs from local farms where I can see the chickens running around.

Dairy products are better tolerated by some people than others. We tell mothers to breast-feed babies in part because a mother's milk contains chemical messengers that direct the baby's development. Cow's milk has chemical messages meant only for calves. It is, consequently, no surprise that cow's milk commonly promotes migraines, nasal allergies, asthma, sinus problems, eczema, and rashes. If you have an autoimmune disorder, you could try stopping cow's milk products for a few months to see if it makes a difference. Goat's milk protein more closely resembles the protein in human milk and may be better tolerated by some people. And there are a variety of milk substitutes available, such as unsweetened almond, coconut, hemp, rice, and soy beverages.

APPETIZING?

Did you know that the US Department of Agriculture has an allowable standard of pus cells in milk? Up to 750 million pus cells are allowed per liter.

The sugar in dairy products, which is called lactose, is a common cause of gas and diarrhea. Some ethnic groups have an intolerance to lactose that develops early in life, and after they are weaned they rarely consume dairy products. Other groups possess the genetic capacity to digest lactose throughout their lives. Still others can tolerate some lactose, some of the time. Occasionally, a person who can digest lactose will develop a problem with it after a bout of diarrhea. I have seen this type of postdiarrhea lactose intolerance last for two years and then go away completely.

In Western developed countries, we eat more protein of animal origin than we need. We would do well to expand our use of easily digested, balanced foods like beans, lentils, and fermented soy. Soy is often a genetically modified food and frequently gets processed to death in the manufacture of newfangled vegetarian foods. I am ambivalent about these textured, soy-protein foods that are designed to look like various cuts of meat. I think it is wiser to look at more traditional versions of soy — fermented miso and cultured tofu, also known as tempeh. These have been food sources for thousands of years. Choose organic soy, since that form is not genetically modified. Genetically modified soy contains a high level of pesticides.

Beans are currently the subject of research, and the findings are proving the old adage "Beans, beans, good for your heart." Anything good for your heart is also good for your blood circulation, which helps healing and reduces pain. Beans are high in antioxidants. They combine protein, fiber, and healthy carbs in one neat, inexpensive package. We should all try to include them in our cooking more often. Using a small amount of animal protein to flavor the dish may satisfy the need for meat but still keep the cost of the meal low.

No matter what you may have heard to the contrary, all varieties of nuts are healthy, including the once-shunned coconut (a fruit really, not a nut).[24] Back in the days when fat was seen as the enemy of good health, we were told to avoid nuts. This was never good advice, and there was never research to support it. Nuts contain protein, fiber, and minerals, as well as healthy oils. It is best to buy raw nuts, because oils in the nuts can become rancid more quickly once they have been roasted.[25] If you roast them yourself, you will know they are fresh. Rancid foods are a source of free radicals that can damage your cells.

Fats and Oils

Eating fat does not make people fat. Fat, as part of a meal, helps your body absorb fat-soluble vitamins and signals the body to feel full and stop eating. In fact, ultra-low-fat diets, especially the ones that are high in high-glycemic carbs, may be responsible for making people lose weight and then gain back even more weight in the common "yo-yo" diet phenomenon.

Olive oil and canola oil are called monounsaturated oils. Olive oil is a monounsaturated omega-9 oil, which contains healthy antioxidant polyphenols. It has a long tradition of use and is partly responsible for the health benefits of the Mediterranean diet. Canola oil is a newly developed monounsaturated oil, but there are some health concerns associated with its excessive use, which some new studies have associated with heart disease. Most canola is genetically modified.

Cholesterol is a type of fat that comes from animal sources. Because animals are at the top of the food chain, these fats are more likely to contain toxics, many of which are lipophilic, meaning they are attracted to fat. For this reason, it is best to limit the intake of full-fat dairy products and fat from meats. Eating organics will reduce the amount of toxics you get from these foods. For most people, eating foods high in cholesterol, in moderation, does not raise their cholesterol or their risk of cardiovascular disease. The cells in our bodies produce cholesterol, and it is needed for healthy cell membranes. Oxidative stress, and not just the presence of cholesterol, is what causes damage to our arteries.[26]

Hydrogenated oils are oils that have been altered to give them a different texture. Many vegetable shortening and margarines have been hydrogenated, and they form trans fats, a source of oxidative stress. Hydrogenated oils have been shown to increase triglycerides, bad cholesterol, total cholesterol, and the risk of cardiovascular disease.

Oils become rancid quickly after heating. They can also deteriorate at high temperatures and form trans fats.[27] Some oils can tolerate higher temperatures before they deteriorate. These oils include coconut oil and some nut oils. All oils are healthier when not heated, and it is best to avoid frying anything at high temperatures.

Essential Fatty Acids

Omega-3 and omega-6 polyunsaturated fatty acids are essential for good health. We need to get them from our food because we cannot make them. They are important to the functioning of every human system, and if properly balanced in our bodies, they ben-efit the immune and inflammation systems. The North American diet is generally too high in omega-6 and deficient in omega-3. Linoleic acid is the main type of omega-6 in American diets and in those of Westernized countries, and when consumed in excess, it promotes inflammation.[28] The omega-3s are alpha-linolenic acid, which comes from plants such as flax, and docosahexa-enoic acid and eicosapentaenoic acid, which come from fish, organic free-range eggs, and grass-fed beef. These omega-3s promote anti-inflammatory pathways. The imbalance of omega-3 in rela-tion to omega-6 contributes to long-term inflam-matory diseases, such as heart disease, cancer, asthma, arthritis, pain, and depression. Primrose oil, borage oil, and organ meats contain an anti-inflammatory omega-6 fatty acid called gamma-linolenic acid, which increases dihomo-gamma-linolenic acid and stimulates an anti-inflammatory pathway.[29]

BALANCING ACT

Generally, omega-6s are proinflammatory and promote the chronic degenerative diseases, while omega-3s, espe-cially docosahexaenoic acid and eicosapenta-enoic acid, are anti-inflammatory and, as a result, protective. But we need a healthy bal-ance of both.

Sweets, Treats, and Beverages

As I mentioned earlier, when working with patients on their diets, I try to add healthy products before I take away the less healthy ones. There are a few exceptions. I strongly urge all patients to immediately stop consuming soda pop, aspartame, and sucralose.

Soda pop is packed with high-fructose corn syrup (HFCS), a sweetener made from corn. Over the past fifty years, it has been added to all sorts of foods, both sweet and savory. Its ubiquity has become astounding. Look for it on labels and avoid it. HFCS raises blood sugar and causes fatty liver, a condition of abnormal deposits of fat in the liver. It is associated with insulin resistance and converts to fat more easily than other sugars. HFCS also increases lactic and uric acids and induces mineral loss through the kidneys. It adds empty calories and much of it contains mercury, a highly toxic heavy metal. A 2009 study found significant mercury contamination in 50 percent of the HFCS sampled.[30] I talk more about mercury in chapter 10.

Worse than HFCS is sucralose.[31] A zero-calorie sweetener, it was devised in a lab in Great Britain by two scientists who were trying to make chlorinated pesticides. They came up with an organochlorine, which is in the same chemical family as dichlorodiphenyltrichloroethane (better known as DDT), and one of them tasted it by accident. Sucralose is the active ingredient listed in many of the packet sweeteners. These sweeteners also contain four calories' worth of sugar as filler, though the packets may not indicate this. Aspartame is the other major zero-calorie sweetener. When heated to 86° Fahrenheit, aspartame breaks down into formaldehyde, most commonly used for preserving corpses, and methanol, a highly toxic alcohol. Normal body temperature is 98.6°.

I recommend that my patients try natural, healthier alternatives to these artificial sweeteners, such as stevia, raw honey, wood sugars like xylitol, and even coconut sugar or, for nondiabetics, regular sugar. Stevia is a sweet leaf and is a healthy, zero-calorie sweetener. Some people can detect a bitter aftertaste in it, but it now comes in a nonbitter version. Xylitol is a wood alcohol and is considered a safe sweetener, one that may also offer some protection for dental enamel.

Even though these natural sweeteners do offer some health benefits, all sweeteners, and especially xylitol and regular sugar, should be taken in small amounts. We would all do well to consume fewer sweets…

The average North American eats 150 pounds of sugar each year. Two hundred years ago, it was only 2 pounds per year.[32] Sugar is as addicting as cocaine and triggers the same reward center of the brain,[33] and is often hidden in processed foods where you would not suspect it — for example, in processed meats, low-fat peanut butter, and supposed-to-be-good-for-you cereals. Most people are born with a preference for or against sweets, but people can also condition their taste buds to crave a high level of sweetness. You can reset your taste buds by eliminating all sweets for a week or two. Who knows, you might not actually prefer four spoonfuls of sugar in that cup of coffee. Everything that was said earlier about high-glycemic foods holds true for sugar, which spikes your blood sugar and leads to carb cravings. It is best to tone down our need for sweet tastes in general. The taste itself, even if the sweetener contains zero calories, may trigger the reaction in our brains that raises our insulin level and sends us off on the glycemic roller coaster.[34]

Chocolate

I always said I consumed chocolate because of a nutrient deficiency. At first, I thought it might be magnesium, then manganese. We now know that it contains antidepressant-like compounds and the potent antioxidants called flavanols. I am finally exonerated. Chocolate is a health food! But only if the chocolate has a high cocoa content (70 percent or higher) and is consumed in moderation. In one study, researchers found that patients suffering from high blood pressure who took a regular dose of dark chocolate over a period of fifteen days saw a reduction in blood pressure, lower total cholesterol, less bad cholesterol, and improved insulin sensitivity.[35] A small amount — probably an ounce or two — of high-cocoa-content chocolate can be a healthy treat. Milk, however, deactivates the antioxidants in chocolate, so milk chocolate is not recommended.

There have been recent reports of lead contamination in chocolate and cocoa. Lead is another highly toxic heavy metal, which I discuss in chapter 10. While the source of the lead has not been discovered, cocoa pods

were found to be free of it, so investigators suspect that environmental contamination might be occurring on the way to the processing plants.

Coffee

Caffeine and coffee are controversial. I am more prone to pay attention
to positive research about coffee because I love it so much. Nevertheless, I do follow my own advice and limit myself to no more than one
cup per day. In addition, every few months I take a break from coffee
consumption for at least two weeks. Coffee and caffeine can interfere
with sleep and may be associated with fluctuat-
ing blood sugar levels. Drinking decaffeinated
coffee does not totally solve the problems. First,
there is still some caffeine in decaf, and second,
coffee, whether decaf or regular, has substances
that irritate the stomach and cause heartburn.

>> **COFFEE FACTETTES**
>>
>> Americans consume
>> over 300 million cups
>> of coffee per day, as
>> reported by CBS in
>> 2009.[36]
>>
>> Coffee is the
>> second-most-traded
>> commodity in the world,
>> behind petroleum.[37]

If you have pain or muscle problems, you
should limit yourself to five or six cups per week.
Caffeine interferes with the movement of calcium
and glucose in and out of your muscle cells and
may increase the secretion of adrenaline. The
wide fluctuations in blood sugar that may be associated with caffeine can make you gain weight and
may contribute to adrenal fatigue. A coffee habit of more than one cup
per day has been associated with elevated estrogen levels, which can affect
many functions in the body, including the tendency to gain weight around
the middle. At the same time, coffee has recently been shown to contain
powerful antioxidants. Caffeine has a half-life of 7.5 hours. This means that
half of the caffeine is still in your system after 7.5 hours. More research is
needed on the subject but, in the meantime, moderation is best.

Tea

Tea (black, green, and white) contains flavonoids called polyphenols. A
powerful group of polyphenols in tea are called catechins, which enhance

your immune system. The immune-system cells of tea drinkers attack germs five times faster than those of coffee drinkers. Tea drinkers have a lower incidence of cancer, and tea may help prevent heart disease. There is research on Alzheimer's and other neurodegenerative diseases that suggests all teas, especially green tea, have a protective effect. Green tea can protect the pancreas, reducing the sugar produced by the liver and making your cells more sensitive to insulin. Matcha, a Japanese green tea, is being studied for its many health benefits. There are no pain studies on tea, but since the mechanisms of inflammation and oxidative stress are the same for these chronic diseases as they are for pain, it can't hurt to drink tea and it probably helps.

The caffeine in tea causes a gentler stimulus than coffee does,[38] and consequently, when the stimulant effect wears off, you are likely to feel less fatigued. Tea does not interfere with sleep as much as coffee does, and it provokes less stomach irritation for most people. Nevertheless, some people are extraordinarily sensitive to caffeine from any source and cannot tolerate coffee or tea.

Decaffeinated teas still contain catechins. Herbal teas are not made from tea leaves and may have other benefits specific to the herbs they are made with. It is important to distinguish between decaffeinated tea made from tea leaves, but with most of the caffeine removed, and herbal teas made with herbs and flowers that never contained caffeine.

Soda

There is nothing redeeming about soda. It is full of empty calories, as sugar or artificial and potentially harmful sweeteners and many other chemicals. The diet varieties are the worst. Manufacturers have recently tried to suggest health benefits in soda by adding vitamins. In fact, these added vitamins cause chemical reactions that increase the level of benzene, a highly toxic and carcinogenic petroleum product, in the beverage.[39]

It has been shown that soda disrupts appetite. Our brain does not know how to deal with the calories in these drinks, so instead it ignores them. This leads to overeating. People who drink soda gain extra weight.

For a soda substitute, use carbonated spring water and flavor it with natural juice, not from concentrate. Both pomegranate and blueberry juice have antioxidant properties. If you have no problems with caffeine, drink iced tea. If caffeine is an issue, then try decaffeinated or herbal iced tea. Teas are usually not a problem for most people and, as I mentioned earlier, are high in flavonoids, polyphenols, and catechins.

Water: Purification, Filters, and Alkaline

Some of our municipal water supplies contain heavy metals and chemicals, including pesticides and drug residues — from birth control pills, blood pressure medications, mood-altering drugs, and other drugs. The long-term consequences of consuming these has never been studied, and while waiting for studies to be done, I recommend filtering your water. There are many filtration systems on the market at various prices. A simple carbon filter can be attached to your kitchen faucet or placed in a pitcher. It will filter out heavy metals and chlorine. A reverse osmosis system will filter out heavy metals, most organic pollutants, and detergents.[40] A distiller will filter out almost everything, including all the trace minerals we need. You can add those trace minerals back into the water by using mineral drops. Check out the costs and specifications of the different types of filters and buy the best one you can afford. This technology is rapidly improving.

Alkaline water is another option. Many of my patients have reported they feel better drinking it. Natural spring water from the earth is mostly alkaline. Although I am unaware of studies showing any health benefit from drinking alkaline water, alkalinizing your body by eating a lot of vegetables and fruits has been shown to be healthy.

Wine, Beer, and Spirits

There are beneficial antioxidants in wine — red wine, especially. Research on alcoholic beverages, however, is still insufficient and doesn't answer some troubling questions. While overall data indicate that people who drink moderately have a decreased risk of heart disease, we still don't know exactly why. In addition, it seems that women who drink even one glass of wine a day have an increased risk of breast cancer. Red wine has resveratrol and other antioxidants that have been associated with the benefits of the Mediterranean diet.

Drink in moderation only. If you need to drink every day, you have a problem. Alcohol is a toxin and it stresses your liver. Women are more prone to liver disease from drinking than men — meaning it takes fewer drinks for women to develop liver disease. It's not fair, but that's life.

Fermented Foods

Many newfangled things in our environment threaten our probiotics. These threats include antibiotics, heavy metal contaminants, high-glycemic foods, and estrogen-like compounds from plastics, petroleum products, and pesticides. Luckily, many fermented foods contain probiotics and prebiotics. Some examples are sauerkraut, pickles, yogurt, kimchi, chutneys, and kefir.

Herbs and Spices

Spices can be the bark, seed, or fruit of a plant. Many spices have health benefits, and I discuss some of them in chapter 7, the supplements chapter. Herbs are generally the leafy green parts of a plant. Herbs also have benefits, specifically to your digestion and metabolism. Additionally, many herbs are anti-inflammatories, antioxidants, or anti-infectives and are useful for treating pain.

Rosemary oil and leaves are potent vasodilators, meaning they cause blood vessels to expand. They also have anti-inflammatory and antioxidant properties. Rosemary, whether eaten as part of your diet or absorbed through your skin by soaking in a bath with rosemary oil, helps to promote good circulation.

Ginger is a powerful anti-inflammatory and is useful for treating pain.[41] It fights inflammation in the body in many different ways.[42] It is also a digestive aid and an effective antinauseant, and it reduces mucus production in the sinuses and the respiratory system. Ginger can be eaten raw or cooked. I peel my ginger and keep it in a jar of sherry in the fridge. I recommend chopping it up and using it in stir fries, coconut dishes, and tea. If you leave chopped ginger in a pitcher of water in the fridge, it makes an invigorating cold beverage.

Turmeric too is in the ginger family. Curcumin is the most active ingredient in turmeric, and sometimes the two names are used interchangeably. Turmeric is best absorbed if mixed with black pepper and oil, as it is in curry. Turmeric has two dozen anti-inflammatory qualities and is good for treating pain.[43] It is also useful in treating arthritis and is currently being researched for Alzheimer's prevention. The journal *Alternative and Complementary Therapies* published a review of hundreds of studies and concluded that "turmeric appears to outperform many pharmaceuticals in its effects against several chronic debilitating diseases, and does so with virtually no adverse side effects."[44]

Cinnamon is another powerful medicinal spice. One-half teaspoon of cinnamon per day can reduce blood sugar, triglycerides, and cholesterol. There is an insulin-like compound in cinnamon that helps sugar enter muscle cells. In muscle cells, sugar is used to produce energy, unlike in fat cells, where it is stored as fat.[45] This is helpful for everyone, but especially so for people with type 2 diabetes.

Some Specific Diets

The suggestions below are different ways of organizing and thinking about the foods you eat. I have also listed some specialized diets for specific health problems.

The Mediterranean Diet

The foods typically eaten by Mediterranean peoples include ample fruits, vegetables, beans, nuts, rice, and pasta. Olives grow abundantly in the region, and olives and olive oil play a big role in food preparation. The

Mediterranean diet features relatively little red meat but usually includes fish and shellfish. Red wine is also part of meals in the region. People who eat this diet appear to have lower rates of cardiovascular disease, even though they eat saturated fats in the form of butter and whole-fat cheeses. When judging the diet, however, it is important to also look at the traditional southern European relationship to food. Most food is bought fresh, and mealtime is a time to focus on the enjoyment of the meal and the company. Many of the French buy a fresh baguette from the bakery, twice a day. They buy only enough bread for a meal or two. Unfortunately, some of this reverence for food is changing as Europeans adopt North American bad habits. The movement called Slow Food began in Italy and is growing in popularity in North America. It promotes old-fashioned values in food preparation and meal enjoyment. There are now some Slow Food restaurants in major cities.[46]

Alkaline Diet

Acids and bases are measured by their pH level. A pH of 7.0 is neutral, meaning it is neither basic (also called alkaline) nor acidic. Anything higher than 7.0 is alkaline, while anything lower is acidic. The pH of our skin is supposed to be around 5.0, meaning it's acidic, while the pH of our blood is ideally 7.5; we have an acidic shell around an alkaline core. In the 1960s, manufacturers suddenly realized that the soaps and cosmetics we were using on our skin and hair were highly alkaline and, as a result, were causing irritation and rashes. Since then, advertisers have conditioned us to look for "pH-balanced" products.

On the other hand, we are still being sold processed, high-glycemic foods that disturb our internal pH level and make our core too acidic. We do not hear as much about this pH disruption because, so far, there are no incentives for advertisers to teach us about it. While pH-balanced skin and hair products can be sold for more than others, bags of beans and broccoli lack the profit margins and addictive qualities of processed foods. A diet rich in fruits, vegetables, and beans and other legumes creates a healthy, alkaline environment inside your body.

But while most of the internal chemical reactions that keep our metabolism running smoothly work better when we are alkaline, too much alkalinity, like too much acidity, is corrosive and damaging. Fortunately, overly alkaline systems are rare and usually only happen because of particular diseases that need medical attention. It is, however, common for people to be too acidic because of bad food habits.[47] If you are in pain, it is important to learn about an alkaline diet. An alkaline diet contains lots of vegetables, seeds, nuts, and whole grains. It can contain some fish, natural yogurt, cheese, and fruit (believe it or not, citrus fruits are allowed), and minimal sugar, white flour, processed foods, dairy, and meat.[48]

Gluten-Free Diet

Gluten is a protein in wheat, rye, barley, kamut, and spelt.[49] Buckwheat is not related to wheat and contains no gluten. There are certified gluten-free oats, but most forms of oats contain gluten because of cross-contamination in the processing.[50]

Classic celiac disease (CD) is a genetic predisposition to develop damage in the bowel when eating gluten. For sufferers of the disease, even trace amounts of gluten can severely damage the lining of the small intestine. CD affects 1 percent of the population, and most people who have it don't know it. It can masquerade as many other conditions, including chronic pain and other autoimmune disorders, and it can cause a variety of diseases, including cancer.

There is some confusion about the difference between CD and the more common gluten sensitivity (GS). A recent study on the two conditions found that the two diseases are very different.[51] Nevertheless, whether individuals suffer from CD or GS, they benefit from a gluten-free diet, and both CD and GS, if ignored, can lead to body-wide inflammation and the development of diseases and unexplained pain. People with the genetic profile for CD or GS, and those with antibodies against gluten, need to avoid gluten, even those whose bowels are not yet damaged.

There are tests for CD and GS. The old standard has been bowel biopsies, which are used to prove damage to the lining of the small intestine. There are also blood tests, stool tests, and now even tests for the genes that cause the condition.

The health consequences of CD and GS are potentially severe. They include anemia, arthritis, bone loss, depression, infertility, seizures, pain, numbness, and a predisposition to diabetes and lymphoma. Sometimes I find gluten intolerance in patients who have difficult-to-control migraines, pain, or body-wide stiffness, which always looks to me like someone trapped inside their own body.

The most typical CD symptom is diarrhea, while the most typical GS symptoms are recurrent skin problems that are hard to diagnose. Your skin is your largest detoxification organ, and when toxics leave your body through it, rashes are often the result. I have seen countless unexplained skin rashes that were a result of negative reactions to food in general. These skin problems are often diagnosed as eczema, dermatitis, or "sensitive skin" but have no clear cause.

I have also seen many pain patients who have had neither diarrhea nor skin rashes who have improved on gluten-free diets.

It is necessary for those who are at risk of gluten sensitivity to avoid all forms of gluten. This used to be difficult in North America, because wheat has become ubiquitous in food preparation. Nowadays there are many alternative grains, and more foods are labeled as gluten-free. More restaurants have gluten-free menus, and there are gluten-free bakeries and dining-out clubs for people with gluten intolerance.

A Case of Gluten Sensitivity

George is a forty-three-year-old master carpenter and builder who runs his own small construction company. He has come to see me because he has back pain and is having trouble doing his work. He has had low iron for a number of years and had many tests to discover why, but no reason was found. He has always had trouble keeping on weight, even as a child. He has a lot of cramping in his gut and bowel gas, and sometimes has loose bowel movements and at other times constipation. He fell and broke his wrist a few years ago. It healed well. When I examine him, I am surprised that his muscles seem as though they are an undersized set of clothes; they are tight all over his body. He can barely turn his head or tilt it to the side. He can only reach his knees with his fingers when he bends forward. He should be able to reach his toes. His hip, leg, arm, and shoulder muscles are all too tight to allow for normal movement. George's family cooks most of their meals at home, and he does not eat junk food. He loves bread, though. He takes no vitamins.

I tell him I'm not sure what is wrong with him, but that I suspect he has a problem with his metabolism or immune system, which would explain such widespread tightness. He has been so focused on back pain that he has not noticed how generally tight his body is; but when he thinks about it, he realizes that he is weaker than he had been and that there are things he is now too inflexible to do. He has learned to live with the idiosyncrasies of his bowel and thought everyone had bowels that behaved that way.

I send off blood samples to be tested for vitamin B, C, and D levels, for iron levels, and for CD and GS. I also do a test for inflammation. He has recently had a physical checkup and blood tests for all the regular things, like liver function, kidney function, and blood count. I tell him to stop all gluten, to start taking vitamin D and magnesium, and to add omega-3 fish oils in high doses. I will see him again in two weeks, when I have his tests back. I also suggest he try the technique of therapy known as Gunn intramuscular stimulation, also called Gunn IMS, which uses acupuncture needles to release tight bands in muscles called trigger points. It also works along the spine to release the muscles there.

George has two sessions of Gunn IMS by the time his blood work comes back. He is feeling a little looser, and his back pain is improving, but he is still tight overall. His blood work shows low iron and low vitamin B, C, and D. His gluten intolerance tests came back showing he has GS.

George stays on a strict gluten-free diet. Over the next several months, he continues with exercise, massage, and Gunn IMS. Six months after his diagnosis, his back pain is much better and he is starting to regain his flexibility.

The Specific Carbohydrate Diet

In the 1950s, Elaine Gottschall researched and promoted dietary treatments of severe intestinal problems after finding that this approach healed her daughter's severe case of ulcerative colitis, a common inflammatory bowel disease, which was unresponsive to any of the standard medical management. She wrote a book called *Breaking the Vicious Cycle*. Her diet eliminates all grains and many legumes. It may be seen by some as extreme; but for those with severe disease, it can heal their gut and spare them the surgical removal of parts of their colon. To me, a diet, no matter how restrictive, seems less extreme than surgery. Over the years, I have had many patients come to me with pain complaints, sometimes in their back, neck, or shoulders, and sometimes due to abdominal or pelvic pain. Many have had bowel symptoms, including diarrhea, blood in their stool, and less specific complaints. Many of them were eventually diagnosed with inflammatory bowel disease or the less severe irritable bowel syndrome. When less-restricted diets did not help these patients, I suggested the Gottschall plan. Most of them benefited from this approach and were able to minimize their use of prescription medications and avoid surgeries. Some bowel conditions can be life threatening, and you should work with medical supervision if you take this route.

Nightshade-Free Diet

The nightshade family consists of tomatoes, potatoes, eggplants, bell peppers, and chili peppers. Tobacco and belladonna also belong to this group. Black and white peppercorns are not nightshades. Nightshades acidify the body. Veterinarians were the first to discover that nightshades can cause pain and arthritic changes in animals. Some people react the same way. These people respond well to a nightshade-free diet, which is a diet that completely excludes the nightshade food group, with no exceptions. Individuals may need to stick with the diet for at least six months before seeing results. Be aware, the nightshade-free diet forbids almost all prepared sauces, because they contain some kinds of peppers.

Blood-Type Diets

Historically, different eating patterns developed in geographical areas based on the foods that were available at the time. For our early ancestors, having the genes to digest food that was available in the region where they lived gave them a survival advantage. Blood-type diets (a different one for each of the four blood types) arose from this idea. In theory, your blood type reflects your ability to digest certain foods and not others. Some people do well by eating according to their blood type, but for many this diet is not the answer. The problem is that most of us are no longer pure products of our ancestral lands. Our predecessors migrated and intermarried, and the way in which our bodies process foods today is polygenic, meaning it entails many genes and not just our blood-type genes. Of course, it would be useful to do a test to determine exactly which types and quantities of foods each of us needs for optimal health, but such tests don't yet exist. So we need another approach to figuring out what works for our systems. *Nutrigenomics* is the term used to describe how our genetic makeup reacts with the foods we eat. Nutrigenomics is a key part of functional medicine — a branch of integrative medicine that focuses on the ideal function of our bodies.

Elimination and Four-Day Rotation Diets

These diets need to be carefully tailored to the individual and supervised in order to be helpful. You may either eliminate or rotate families of foods. For example, if you are eliminating legumes, then you have to avoid peanuts as well because they are related. In an elimination diet, you reduce the number of foods you eat to a few that you are pretty certain you tolerate well. Then you gradually reintroduce new foods about once a week. In a four-day rotation diet you eat a food from one food family no more often than every four days. These diets are usually needed by people who are sensitive to a large number of foods, and the diets can help clarify what they can safely eat.

Other Alternative Diets

There are countless alternative diets, including the Nutritional Type diet, macrobiotic diet, Gut and Psychology Syndrome diet, and many others.

If you have chronic pain, it is worth experimenting with different diets to see if they make a difference. I have personally seen the alkaline, grain-free, gluten-free, specific-carbohydrate, elimination, and four-day rotation diets all used successfully. When you decide to try one of these diets, do not approach it with the attitude that you have just decided to give up a particular item forever. It makes it more difficult if you start with the attitude that you will never taste, for example, spaghetti sauce or ketchup again. Instead, approach the diet as a limited-time experiment. For some diets, you can quickly see a change in your health, meaning in as little time as a month or so. For others, you must persist for as long as six months, which is true of the nightshade- and gluten-free diets. Once you start to see positive results, you will be more motivated to make any necessary lifelong changes. At that point, people often perceive the elimination of the foods not as a loss but as an unexpected gift of health.

For more information about diets, see the Resources section.

Advice for Busy People

If you do not have time to shop and cook proper meals, I suggest taking some shortcuts that will allow you to still eat well. Buy bags or trays of precut vegetables and keep them in the fridge with a healthy dip like humus, salsa, or tzatziki. If you like to cut up your own vegetables, I recommend taking one day — Sunday, for example — to buy, wash, and cut your veggies for the rest of the week. When you get home from work and are rushing to prepare dinner, take out the veggies and the dip and nibble while you cook. If you have kids, they will dig in too. You may end up having three to four servings of vegetables before you even get to eat dinner. It's a snack that is low calorie and high in fiber, minerals, and enzymes — there is no downside. Having cut-up veggies also makes it easy to take a container or bag of them to work. In addition, keep nuts, seeds, and balanced protein bars in your desk, purse, or briefcase. That way, you will have a healthy alternative to the donuts or chips that may tempt you over the course of the day.

I frequently cook more food than I know I will eat in a meal, and I freeze the extra food in glass containers with snap-on lids. That way, I can have a nutritious meal even on days that I have no time to cook. I really enjoy vegetable soups, sometimes pureed and other times with vegetable chunks. When I am making vegetable juice with my juicer, I often save some of the pulp and add lentils, water, and an organic bouillon cube and make a healthy, high-fiber soup. The soup makes a fabulous dinner when served with a whole grain bread and cheese (gluten-free bread and goat cheese for me). For extra protein and flavor, you can also add a piece of meat to the soup while it's cooking.

Foods don't need elaborate preparation to be wholesome and tasty. Try a simple fish dinner, for example. A lot of people are nervous about cooking fish, but a good-tasting fish dish is really not difficult to prepare. I like to grill fish, sauté it, bake it, or broil it. A foolproof way for beginners to cook fish is to use a frying pan and a lid. Add a tablespoon of olive oil or butter and then the fish. Heat over a low heat and then add some wine (½ cup) and soy sauce (1 tbsp). Add ground pepper. If you want to get fancier, you can sauté some onions and ginger in the oil before you add the fish. Cook covered for five to ten minutes, depending on the thickness of the fish. If the liquid boils off before your fish is cooked, add a little water and turn down the heat. You can change the flavors of your fish by using different liquids and spices. You can use coconut milk with ginger, onion, garlic, and cinnamon, or add some lemon juice with pepper. This recipe will always be moist and tasty.

Love Your Food

Eating has the potential to be one of the great pleasures in life. It's the satisfaction of a primitive instinct, and it should be a sensual experience of vision, touch, smell, and taste. Traditionally, eating has also been important for maintaining the social fabric of society; a meal was a place to make friends and spend time with families. Nowadays, eating has become something we just have to do, like filling the gas tank in our car. And sometimes it takes even less time.

- Try enjoying your food by using some adventurous approaches.
- Make a rainbow on your plate using the natural colors of food.
- Focus on the taste of your food by eating slowly. Savor each flavor, and stop before you are full — tease yourself.
- Don't do other things while you eat; focus only on eating.
- Have family-time meals. Make conversation and tell stories about what each family member learned that day or feels grateful for.
- Listen to your favorite music while you eat.
- Be a daredevil — take a risk and try a new food. Try a small amount of that new food on five separate occasions before you decide if you do or don't like it. That was the rule for my kids, and they ended up liking most things they tried.

CHAPTER 5

RESOLVE STRESS AND DISSOLVE PAIN
The Mind-Body Solution

Mind doesn't dominate body; it becomes body. Body and mind are one.
I see the process of communication we have demonstrated, the flow
of information throughout the whole organism, as evidence that the body is
the actual outward manifestation, in physical space, of the mind.

— CANDACE PERT, *Molecules of Emotion*

Hippocrates is the earliest recorded physician and medical philosopher, and we credit him with founding Western medicine. He practiced and philosophized over two thousand years ago. He was a holistic healer, which means he treated patients as a whole and not as a collection of parts, where each part could be treated as though it were separate from the others. Holism suggests the body cannot be separated from the mind and spirit. In general, the ancient healers, including aboriginal Americans, Africans, and others, were holistic.

Science took a turn away from holism during the seventeenth century, when René Descartes, often regarded as the father of modern philosophy, published a treatise endorsing dualism. It is perhaps no coincidence that this new attitude toward medicine was directly in line with church doctrine of the time — the church had severe ways of influencing scientific philosophers.[1] In any case, Descartes's ideas pushed science down the path of a mind-body split. This left the mind and spirit in the unchallenged domain of the church while allowing medical science to investigate the despirited body.

This focus on the physical body led to countless useful discoveries. During the time after Descartes, we learned a lot about anatomy, physiology, the heart, and circulation. These were important discoveries that gave us the foundation for our understanding of the human body. But the human is more than the sum of the body's physical parts, just as music is more than the sum of the instruments used to play it. Since Descartes, allopathic medicine has focused almost exclusively on the physical body, and the interconnection between the mind and body has been only rarely discussed.

Looking at the body as a machine has limited our ability to understand some of the complex workings of our system. Dualism has kept us from seeing that all conditions affect both mind and body. Over the past forty years, scientific discoveries have pushed medicine back toward holism. New research studies have shown us that the mind and the body use the same system of communication. Holism has been reborn as mind-body medicine.

To better understand the body-mind,[2] let's review some of the scientific evidence for a body-wide communication system. The gut has 100 million neurons, or nerve cells — enough for a small brain. It produces 80 percent of our melatonin, which we used to think came only from the pineal gland in the brain, and it produces 80 percent of our serotonin, which is supposed to be the brain chemical that improves our mood. Why does our gut make chemicals associated with brain function? We don't yet really know, but maybe it explains why we have "gut feelings."

The human heart is best known as the pump that circulates blood to every part of the body. It also has between forty thousand and ninety thousand nerve cells, puts out an electromagnetic field that spreads eight feet around us in all directions,[3] and makes and releases both norepinephrine, which is a stress hormone and neurotransmitter, and dopamine, another brain chemical. This is fascinating because every language and culture has expressions involving emotions and instincts associated with the heart. It seems the heart is way more than just a sophisticated pump, but we have unanswered questions about the heart's other functions. What can we perceive from the electromagnetic field of others? Is this what we refer to when we say someone has a real presence — an energy we like or don't like? The neurotransmitters in the heart are the same ones known to create emotional responses in our brain. Are they responsible for the age-old words *heartfelt*, *downhearted*, and *heart-break*, or the age-old saying "Follow your heart"?

The immune system defends the body from foreign invaders, such as infections. Lymphocytes are types of immune cells called white blood cells. They can produce natural painkillers and the stress hormone ACTH. This hormone usually comes from the endocrine system, which is a system of several hormone-producing glands, including the thyroid and adrenal glands. Monocytes are another type of white blood cell, and they have receptors for every known neurotransmitter, the chemical messengers once thought to be mainly brain communication molecules. It turns out that when we are under stress, monocytes can even produce those same neurotransmitters!

So it seems our immune cells are talking to the glands in our endocrine system using brain language. Most of the immune system is also closely connected with the gut. In fact, 70–80 percent of the immune system lies beside the small intestine.[4] The gut also makes chemicals that talk to the brain and are associated with our thoughts, feelings, and moods. Of course, all the parts of our nervous system are connected to one another too.[5] These connections allow our mind, our brain, and our body to each influence the function of the others. It turns out that there is a body-wide communication system that uses the same system of messengers, and all of our parts communicate with and influence all the other parts. It is not that we "think" ourselves into pain or out of it, or that we make up our problems. What we think can change how we experience the problems we have and how the body reacts. The reaction goes from mind to brain to body and back again.

There is just one interconnected and complicated system that uses the same methods of communication throughout our mind, brain, and body. This information is useful in treating all forms of illness but is especially important in pain medicine. To live with less pain, we must learn how our body interacts with the rest of the body-mind and learn ways to help this complicated system help itself. The field of mind-body medicine grew out of these ideas.

Stress

The main focus of mind-body medicine is stress. As I explain in this chapter, stress is not always a negative thing — it actually keeps us alive. But when stress is more than we can handle, it can chip away at our health.

Stress changes how we experience pain. For example, any young child knows that mommy's kiss on a boo-boo makes it feel better. The kiss itself may not heal the boo-boo faster, but it soothes the child, which changes his experience of suffering. The kiss may even help healing by reducing stress that promotes inflammation and interferes with healing. As we grow older, if we are lucky, we learn ways to soothe ourselves.

Let's look at how the nervous system deals with stress and how stress affects pain. There are two main subdivisions of the nervous system. The central nervous system is made up of the brain and spinal cord. The peripheral nervous system is the part of the nervous system outside of the brain and the spinal cord. It too is divided into two parts: the somatic system and the autonomic system. The somatic system regulates what we control through the muscles of our skeleton — like moving our arms and legs. The autonomic system has two parts, called the sympathetic and parasympathetic systems. They regulate functions we regard as automatic, like blood pressure control, heart rate, breathing, bowel function, and others. It turns out that we can learn to control some of the autonomic functions too, by learning techniques that I discuss here. The sympathetic system dominates us when we are stressed, and it causes inflammation. The parasympathetic system dominates when we are relaxed. It secretes acetylcholine from the nervous system, which counteracts inflammation. Ideally there should be a balance between the sympathetic and parasympathetic systems.

The sympathetic system and its stress response are necessary for everyday life.[6] Without it, we would not have enough blood pressure to stand up without fainting. When we get stressed, we have an acute stress response, which is also called a "fight or flight" reaction. Your body might have an acute stress response if you wake up in the middle of the night to the sound of a window breaking; your body goes into an emergency mode that quickly decides on the best way to survive the situation. Your brain and body coordinate and are ready to spring into action. In this case, an adaptive stress response may help keep you alive. If we see stress as a challenge that we can handle, it energizes us. But when stress feels overwhelming, it's called distress, which has a negative effect on our health and our response to pain and illness.[7] Some interesting research shows that distress can speed up the aging process by affecting little structures in our cells called telomeres. These structures allow our cells to multiply. Every time a cell multiplies, its telomeres get a little shorter. When telomeres get too short, our cells cannot duplicate, and eventually they die off. We need our cells to multiply in order to heal ourselves and keep our organs in good working order. It turns out that a person who has distress gets shorter telomeres compared to a person who just has stress. The two people may have identical stresses in their lives — the only difference is that one of them finds those stresses overwhelming. This is just one example of the direct health benefits that come from learning to judge our level of stress and ways to manage it.

Before we go on to learn some helpful methods to control stress, it is important to understand a little more about how the stress system changes the functions of the other systems in our body. There are two types of stress — acute stress and chronic stress. Acute stress, as mentioned earlier, is usually short-lived but severe. Our response to it — our fight-or-flight reaction — comes from the primitive predator-prey relationship. Both predator and prey, lion and gazelle, have the same response to acute stress. When a lion hunts a gazelle, adrenal glands in both animals release two major classes of mediators: glucocorticoids (cortisol — a hormone) and catecholamines (adrenaline and noradrenaline — neurotransmitters). These substances then trigger a cascade of effects on a multitude of target cells, causing the release of other hormones and communication molecules. The result is the same in both animals — their digestion and immune-system functions stop, their minds focus sharply on the task at hand, their big muscles get enhanced function, and sugar and fat circulate for energy needs. The run is generally over quickly, leaving either a hungry lion or a dead gazelle. The surviving animal shakes off the stress and its body functions return to normal until the next chase begins.

Chronic stress, on the other hand, is prolonged and not necessarily severe. These days, chronic stress is what we most often mean when we talk about stress. Everyday sources of this stress could be the workplace, an abusive relationship, economically difficult times, uncertainty in the age of terrorism, living in crowded cities, pollution, improper foods, irregular eating habits, or not enough physical activity, to name just a few. But just because chronic stress is common doesn't mean it's natural. Chronic stress is actually a modern phenomenon, and so we have no appropriate primitive response to it. Our body's response to chronic stress is the same as its response to acute stress — our heart rate, blood pressure, and blood sugar go up, our blood flows to our big muscles, our attention focuses so we can respond quickly to possible threats, and sugar and fat are released into the bloodstream so we are ready for action.[8] Other functions that are not needed for immediate survival shut down, including our digestion, sex hormone production, immune system, and circulation to nonessential areas. This stress system, which helps us survive acute stress, makes us sick in the case of chronic stress. Over long periods, the stress response causes inflammation and wear and tear on our system, and it promotes all the chronic diseases that are so common these days — diabetes, heart disease, strokes, and chronic pain.

STRESS AND EMOTIONS

There is a direct connection between stress and your emotions. Stress sharpens the function of the amygdala, which plays a role in your emotional memory, especially fear. The amygdala gets information from the autonomic nervous system and is very sensitive to glucocorticoids. This helps to explain our emotional response to stress, as well as the increased stress levels in those with a history of emotional trauma.

Sadly, people who have been traumatized as children are more likely to have chronic stress and chronic pain syndromes. Moreover, studies have shown that early childhood trauma increases chances of irritable bowel syndrome later in life.[9] In addition, children who have been abused often have higher levels of stress hormones and glucocorticoids in their circulation. Stress hormones and glucocorticoids can change the function and structure of the hippocampus, the part of the brain responsible for long-term memory, by disrupting some of the connections between the nerve cells.

A Case of Chronic Stress

Sharon is on her way to work. She overslept and rushed out without eating, only to find she forgot her briefcase and had to run back for it. This means she missed the 7:18 bus that would get her to the 8:12 train. She arrives at the office at 9:14 instead of 9:00, where she is greeted by her new supervisor, who lectures her on punctuality. When she gets to her desk, she discovers that the coffee cup she left there last evening was knocked over by the cleaning staff and it has left the report for her top client account (due to be delivered at noon) a sticky mess. She is due for a 9:30 meeting in the conference room with all the big bosses, but she now has to produce another copy of all the graphs, charts, and analyses that were in the report. She goes into the meeting twenty minutes late...and this is just the start of Sharon's day. It's full of stress, and her periods of recovery are very brief.

STRESS SIGNATURES

Researchers have noticed that the reactions to stress — that is, responses in heart rate, blood pressure, blood sugar, muscle tension, or other features — of a particular animal or person may be unique to that individual. This may be interesting to consider when looking for solutions to your own pain problem. Can you figure out your pattern? Do your neck, shoulders, and jaw get tight? Do you breathe differently? Does your stomach get sore, or do you have to run to the bathroom a lot? Knowing your pain pattern may help you come up with solutions.

Sharon went to the doctor last week because she was having trouble sleeping and has developed headaches that feel like a band encircling her head. She has started taking an over-the-counter headache medicine, but it gives her heartburn. She has also been gaining weight and sometimes has constipation and other times, diarrhea. Her periods are painful and irregular, and she gets sick all the time. She had a few minutes to describe her symptoms to the doctor, who was writing the prescriptions while she spoke. He told her that her blood pressure is too high and that he was sending her for a test. The prescriptions were for a new headache pill, two kinds of stomach pills, and a sleeping pill. She was told to get a blood test for diabetes. After a brief examination, the doctor left the room — Sharon had been squeezed into his already-packed day. She stared at the prescriptions, feeling more stressed because she did not understand why she needed the drugs and was unsure what was wrong with her. She had questions but no one to ask.

All of Sharon's problems could be caused by chronic stress, and the handful of prescriptions she was given are unlikely to make her feel any better. Chronic stress is likely causing imbalances in Sharon's stress and antistress hormones, which would lead to muscle tension, which would explain her headaches. This would also lead to a lack of a hormone called melatonin, which would explain her trouble sleeping. This hormone imbalance would also cause the heart to pump harder, and the thickening of blood vessels, which would explain her high blood pressure. All of this would naturally affect her immune system too, making her more likely to get sick.

She does not have a healthy diet and may be bingeing on sweets and starches to make up for lost energy, which would cause weight gain. In addition, she may have a problem with her thyroid gland, which would also cause weight gain. As you can see, chronic stress can affect every system in Sharon's body, making it difficult for her to feel healthy and happy. Sharon's story is not that unusual. You probably know people who feel very much as she does.

Stress and Pain: Extreme Examples

Stress changes how we feel pain, in some puzzling ways. There are two extreme examples called stress-induced hyperalgesia and stress-induced analgesia. Stress-induced hyperalgesia happens when people experience more pain as a result of stress. Pain can increase when you are under stress or anticipating pain. Stress-induced analgesia is just the opposite — a lack of pain, as a result of stress. You may have heard of a football player finishing a game on a broken leg. Henry Beecher, a World War II doctor, described stress-induced analgesia in some severely injured soldiers who did not complain about pain while on the battlefield, but who, once safely in the hospital, did complain about the pain from an intravenous needle.

Mind-Body Medicine Solutions

Whether you think you can, or you think you can't — you're right.

— HENRY FORD

Harvard's Herbert Benson described the "relaxation response" when he studied Tibetan monks who could change their body functions, lower their blood pressure and heart rate, and raise their own temperature just by meditating. He even realized that, as a cardiologist, he could sometimes provide better care to his patients by teaching Tibetan Buddhist meditation techniques than by more drastic cardiac interventions. Elizabeth Blackburn showed that we can help our telomeres, those little things that allow our cells to keep multiplying, to recover by using relaxation techniques. In this section I discuss ways in which you can change your body chemistry and change your experience of pain by protecting yourself from distress through the relaxation response. Mind-body techniques can give you a sense of control.

Breathing Techniques

Let's start with breathing. Many traditions associate breath with our life force or vital energy.[10] Hippocrates felt that breath was the most necessary and supreme component in us. Most traditional medical systems, including Traditional Chinese Medicine, Ayurveda, and Native American practices, pay careful attention to how we breathe.[11] They often use breathing techniques to achieve meditation states and deep relaxation. Breath control is a path to spirituality and the mysteries of oneness with forces beyond the self.

In medical school, doctors learn the basics of how the lungs work and about unhealthy changes to breathing. But there are positive aspects of breath and ways to use breathing techniques to better our health. When we are stressed, our breath tends to be shallow. We use only the top part of our lungs and fail to breathe deeply. This leaves stale air trapped in the bottom part of the lungs. Also, when we are stressed, or when we are concentrating on a particular task, sometimes even a sports activity, we may hold our breath. This leaves the blood with insufficient oxygen to deliver to our tissues. As a result, we may become drowsy and confused and experience muscle fatigue. There is research showing that breathing exercises can reduce anxiety, alter heart function, lower blood pressure, reduce the severity of asthma attacks, improve the quality of sleep, and increase energy and mental clarity.[12] Relaxation and meditation that use proper breathing techniques can also relieve pain and improve the quality of sleep.[13] Deep breathing helps to massage internal organs, including the heart, and improve lung capacity. Muscles need oxygen for their metabolic functioning and in order to heal injuries. In addition, good lung capacity is associated with longevity.[14] The best part is that you can do breathing exercises anywhere, with no equipment needed.

Candace Pert, PhD, the well-known researcher who discovered opioid receptors in the brain, has changed our understanding of the molecules of communication called peptides that operate our body-mind. "The peptide-respiratory link is well documented," she writes. "Virtually any peptide found anywhere else can be found in the respiratory center. This peptide substrate may provide the scientific rationale for the powerful healing effects of consciously controlled breath patterns."[15] The ability to change your body and brain chemistry is always just one breath away. Following are some examples of breathing exercises for you to try.

ALTERNATE-NOSTRIL BREATHING

Sit upright in a comfortable position. You will use your right thumb and ring finger to close your nostrils alternately. Put your right ring finger on your left nostril to close the air passage. Breathe in through your right nostril. Pause at the end of a deep inhalation. When you are ready to breathe out, release your index finger and close your right nostril with your thumb and breathe out fully through your left nostril. Pause. Inhale through your left nostril. Press your left nostril closed with your ring finger and release your thumb and breathe out through your right nostril. Continue for as many minutes as you can spare. Each exhale should be about twice as long as the inhale. You might find that this yogic breathing practice calms you, clears your mind, and gives you energy.

UJJAYI

Ujjayi (pronounced oo-ja-EE) is another yogic technique of breathing. Sit comfortably upright. Take a big breath in through your nose and breathe out through your mouth, making the sound *HHHAAA*. Now breathe in and out through your nose but try to make the same *HHHAAA* sound from your throat during both the inhale and the exhale. Breathe in a steady rhythm, spending equal time breathing in and out, while making this sound from your throat. Another way to think of making the sound is to pretend that you are trying to fog up a mirror while breathing out through your mouth. Now make the same sound while breathing through your nose.

THREE-PART BREATH

Sit comfortably upright and breathe through your nose. Before starting the three-part breath, take a few deep cleansing breaths and breathe out as much air as you can, using your stomach muscles to help you. Inhale and feel the breath go into the lowest one-third of your lungs, and feel your belly push out. Pause for a second but don't exhale. Then fill the middle one-third of your lungs and feel your ribs and breastbone expand. Still don't exhale. Then finally fill up the top of your lungs and feel the upper chest expand. Then slowly exhale through your nose in the reverse order: let the air out of the top of your lungs, then the middle, and finally let your belly contract to help you empty the air from the bottom of your lungs. Try to take twice as long to breathe out as to breathe in. You should find a comfortable rhythm for your breathing and not feel strained. Do ten cycles.

Meditation

Meditation is another antidote to the harmful effects of stress. It changes your body chemistry and brings your body rhythms into sync with one another.[16] It can lower your levels of stress hormones, decrease excessive muscle tension, normalize blood pressure, reduce anxiety, and increase pain tolerance. The particular practice called mindfulness-based stress reduction is based on Buddhist meditation techniques and has been studied and made popular by Jon Kabat-Zinn.[17] Research has shown it to be a powerful technique with benefits for patients with chronic pain and anxiety.

There are many different types of meditation. Some use concentration: you focus your attention on only one thing, such as a sound or mantra. Some employ mindfulness: you quiet your mind by excluding outside thoughts and plans, and you focus on the awareness of everything you are experiencing in that moment and from moment to moment. People think of meditation as something they have to sit still for. That appeals to some, but others just don't "have the time" or "get bored." Some forms of meditation involve stillness and some involve movement. "The real meditation," says Kabat-Zinn, "is how you live your life."[18] You can practice using a variety of things: your breath, eating a meal, going for a walk, or a series of movements (as in yoga, qi gong, and tai chi). Any moment in your life can become mindful if you clear your mind of the daily clutter and attend to it: the look on a child's face, the fragrance of a flower, the taste of a meal...

MINDFULNESS MEDITATION

Sit in a comfortable position, either cross-legged on the floor (use pillows to prop up your knees if you need to) or in a chair. Rest your hands comfortably on your knees and take a few deep, cleansing breaths. Close your eyes to limit distraction. Focus on your breathing: breathe in ...breathe out. You may notice that your mind is wandering and thinking about the office or the next chore you must do. Just acknowledge the thought and bring yourself back to focusing on your breathing. Each time your mind wanders, bring it back to your breathing, without judgment. Mindfulness is about being rather than about doing. Do this for ten minutes each day.

WALKING MEDITATION

This is one of my favorites because it combines two things I love to do. You don't have to walk very far. Wear comfortable clothes and shoes. As you step, pay attention to the feeling in your feet as you place your heels on the ground and then roll toward your toes. Your weight shifts, and you are about to put your other foot to the ground and take the next step. Just observe the sensations in your feet, ankles, legs, and hips, and up through your body. Are you swinging your arms? What do they feel like? How does the air feel on your face? Is there a breeze? What can you see? People, flowers, the horizon? Are there noises? Loud ones, like cars and voices? Soft ones, like the air as you brush past? The sound of your footsteps? Your breath? When thoughts of your to-do list come to mind, just acknowledge them and then bring your attention back to your walk.

EATING MEDITATION

Food tastes better when you don't eat quickly — when you give your taste buds a chance to really experience the food. When my three children were young, I used to "inhale" my meals. Mealtime was so rushed that I didn't think I would get to eat if I ate slowly. If I could change that part of history, I would. It was not good for my health, my weight, or my children. I set a bad example for them, and now when I nag them to eat more slowly, they point and say I am a hypocrite. I am trying to eat as many meals as I can mindfully, and I have slowed down my overall pace of eating. I find I enjoy the food more and am satisfied with smaller portions. Try to choose one meal each day during which you eat mindfully.

Take your plate of food and sit down comfortably. Take a moment to look at the colors of the food on your plate. Then smell the aromas of the food. Try to distinguish as many different aromas or just enjoy the blend of them. Take a forkful of food and, before you put it into your mouth, hold it close to your mouth and see if you can already "taste" it. Then slowly put it in your mouth and feel the texture. Begin to chew slowly. You will feel digestive enzymes being released along with saliva to help you digest your food. Chew for twice as long as you ordinarily would. Then swallow and wait a moment before you decide which morsel of food you will pick up next. Choose a different part of the meal, if there is more than one type of food on your plate.

Notice the different aromas, textures, and tastes, and continue eating this way until you are full. Then ask yourself, "How did it feel to eat this way?" Did it change your attitude to the food?

I recently heard of a woman who used to gobble a fast-food burger and fries each lunchtime. After learning about mindful eating, she ate one of those lunches mindfully. After that, she stopped eating fast food because she no longer liked the aroma, texture, and taste, which all seemed acceptable when she used to gobble it down.

GRATITUDE MEDITATION

Focusing on gratitude allows you to open your mind to those things in your life that are good. We all have something to be grateful for: waking up to a new day, a beautiful sunset (or cloud formation if you live in Seattle), having relatives or friends who have touched us, perceiving the beauty of a flower, experiencing the companionship of a pet. In a psychology study, each week for ten weeks people wrote down five things they were grateful for.[19] They were compared to two other groups, one whose members wrote down five burdens from the week, and another whose members simply listed five events. The gratitude group became 25 percent happier than either of the other groups. Perhaps gratitude moves us outside of our ego or makes us feel connected. Whatever the reason, it is a good practice.

Gratitude meditation is easy. As you fall asleep each night review five things you are grateful for. You can combine this with a relaxing breathing exercise or one of the other meditations. Be prepared to be happier over time.

Meditation practices are one way people feel connected to something larger than themselves and appreciate the spiritual aspects of their lives. Many people find that the experience of, and connection to, the mysterious, the sacred, that which is beyond their everyday experience, helps keep their day-to-day stresses in perspective.

Spirituality and Religion

It used to be that the terms *spirituality* and *science* could not appear in the same sentence. There was no room in science for a spiritual self. However, some recent developments in science are changing this paradigm. Now people who talk of spirituality are no longer on the "fringe," and those who deny the importance of the spirit can be accused of not keeping up with the science.

Religion is still a controversial issue for some people. Research shows that people who have a regular religious practice, regardless of which practice it is, live longer and healthier lives. We can suppose that the predictable aspect of a regular religious practice and the calm and meditative aspects of it are responsible for the health benefits.

Other aspects of religion often included in the discussion of spirituality are more controversial, such as intercessory prayer, the practice of having people pray for the health of others. Many studies and papers have been written about it, and so far the jury is still out about its effectiveness, scientifically speaking. But if you are so inclined, do not be discouraged by the lack of science in this delicate area, because as far as we can tell there is no downside. The books of Larry Dossey, MD, report many interesting studies and anecdotal accounts, which make fascinating reading.

One interesting study examined the fMRIs (functional MRIs, which can see changes in brain function) of people being sent distant intentionality, which was defined as healing thoughts sent at a distance by healers. Each pair, the recipient being treated and the therapist sending the distant intentionality, had known each other before and worked together. The person receiving the healing was in the fMRI machine and the therapist was in another place, shielded from all contact with the recipient. The therapist would begin to "treat" the patient at a random time and then stop. The fMRI results were astounding: the fMRIs changed in the patients during the time the distant intentionality was sent. The results were statistically significant, meaning that they could not be explained by chance alone.[20]

We do not know how to account for the findings of the research on spirituality and the Dossey work. Some would dismiss them for that reason. But the sun warmed us and helped us grow food for millions of years before we understood the science that causes the explosions on the sun to radiate life-giving rays to Earth. We should not dismiss data simply because we do not understand it. We can keep an open mind and use those things that are useful to us, as long as they do not cause us harm.

Relaxation Techniques

Guided imagery, autogenic training, biofeedback, and hypnotherapy are all techniques that can enable us to reach deep states of relaxation. As we saw above, it was thought that the autonomic nervous system and things such as heart rate and blood pressure could not be voluntarily controlled. But it turns out that with proper training we can, for example, be trained to slow our heart rate and lower our blood pressure. We can dilate our peripheral blood vessels and make our cold hands warm. This type of training can also be used to control our response to pain and thereby change our experience of pain. All these techniques require practice and have increased benefits with frequent use or training.

GUIDED IMAGERY

This is usually done with a recording or a guide who talks you through the exercise. It is a form of focused attention that leads you along a path of "images," though they need not be only visual images. Some people can see images in their imagination, and others prefer to imagine hearing things, feeling things, or tasting things. It is generally relaxing and often involves mentally going to a safe place of your own choosing. There are many guided-imagery CDs and MP3s on the market. I am going to give you an example of taste imagery. It is best if you have someone read it to you while you are sitting comfortably with your eyes closed.

MY FIRST EXPOSURE

In the mid-1970s, before I went to medical school, I volunteered in the Department of Psychiatry at a veterans' hospital near Los Angeles. We were running a group program for cancer patients using the Simonton guided-imagery methods developed by oncologist Carl Simonton and his wife, Karen. I guess this was my first experience with a mind-body program, even though that label hadn't been invented yet. I was impressed with the methods and the results, but there was barely any science to support it. When I started medical school a few years later, I would not have guessed that I would wholeheartedly come full circle, back to those beginnings.

Imagine you are in a kitchen. Food is cooking quietly on the stove. You go over to the refrigerator and take out a plump, juicy lemon. You hold it in your hand, feeling the coolness. You put it close to your nose and get a faint aroma of lemon through the intact peel. You go over to the counter and take out a cutting board, and with a knife you cut the lemon in half. Some of the juice has spurted out and the aroma of lemon is strong. You see the beads of juice on the cut surface. Then you cut each half again so the lemon is in quarters, and you notice where a seed has been cut through. You pick up one of the quarters and hold it close to your nose and appreciate the lemony smell, then you bring the lemon to your mouth and bite into it.

Are you salivating yet? This is an example of how a mere image in your mind can change your body function. There is no real lemon there, but most people will salivate as if there were.

Autogenic Training

Autogenic training is another relaxation technique that helps you to reduce the effects of stress in your body by taking you through a series of images and affirmations. Mostly the statements address the symptoms of stress and aim at helping you achieve relaxation. There are tapes and therapists who can help with this practice. The scripts vary, but they go something like this. Sit or lie down comfortably. Make sure you are not cold. Repeat each of the following statements three times and try to feel, in your body, the sensation suggested by the words.

I am completely calm.
My arms feel heavy and warm.
My legs feel heavy and warm.
My heartbeat is calm and regular.
My breathing is calm and regular.
My abdomen is warm and comfortable.
My forehead is pleasantly cool.
My neck and shoulders are heavy and warm.
I am at peace.

BIOFEEDBACK

Biofeedback, another relaxation technique, has traditionally used electronic instruments, such as blood pressure monitors and galvanic skin response meters, to aid in the training, but something as simple as biodots, small temperature-sensitive discs applied to the hands, can teach some of the same principles. People can learn to control specific functions; for example, they can increase their blood flow and relieve muscle tension and even migraine headaches.

HYPNOTHERAPY

Hypnotherapy is way to focus attention and achieve a state of deep relaxation. Some people fear hypnosis because they remember the night-club acts where it seemed that people could be made to do things they would not normally do. Unlike in extremes of brainwashing, as seen in spy movies, you are in control when you are hypnotized. Hypnotherapy is often used for pain relief in childbirth and with headaches and other conditions as well.[21]

HUMOR

Humor is a great way to de-stress. People have used humor in tragic theater since the Greek chorus in ancient times. Shakespeare made comic relief a regular part of his tragedies. Comedy helps us cope with the catastrophic. Laughter is infectious, and brain and body chemistry change in response to humor. There is now laughter yoga, which uses nonverbal exercises. Most participants start out pretending to laugh along with the program and usually end up in genuine fits of laughter. Laughter causes some of the same physiological changes as exercise and helps balance the sympathetic and parasympathetic systems.[22] Some research from Norway indicates that humor may prolong life.[23] Norman Cousins, in the autobiographical *Anatomy of an Illness*, explains how humor was his best distraction from pain and helped him recover from a debilitating disease that his doctors had not expected him to survive.[24] In his book he lists funny lines from newspaper want ads that his friends collected for

him. No matter how many times I read them, I am in hysterics. Loretta
Laroche and Patch Adams, MD, are health care professionals who have
turned to laughter and humor in medical settings, and there is an entire
program for medical clowns in Israel called the Dream Doctors. The
Dream Doctors program is a three-year course to train medical clowns
who have become part of the pediatric hospitals around the country.
They are developing a graduate program as well. Patients and health
care personnel state that the Dream Doctors reduce stress and help the
children through traumatic and painful events.

Look at someone who is frowning, then look at someone who has
even a little smile. Does it feel different for you? Who would you rather
be faced with? Remember you have that effect on others when you smile.

SWEARING MAKES YOU FEEL LESS PAIN

A British study suggests that under experimental circumstances, swearing helps to increase pain tolerance. The researchers have speculated
about a variety of mechanisms that may be responsible for this. If you
choose this coping mechanism too often, however, beware of the effects
it has on those around you.

Very negative people I have met puzzled me with their good health
and longevity. Their lives seemed to contradict the science showing that
people with positive attitudes are more likely to be blessed with good
health and long life. The reason swearing works may be illuminated by the
British study of behavior in monkey troops. Some monkeys with negative attitudes who find a way to deflect negative outcomes and blame an
underling actually experience a less harmful stress response, which could
explain why some folks who always find someone else to blame live the
longest.

Pain as a Verb

We have had a look at mind-body practices that can help you deal with
pain, excess stress, anxiety, depression, and even some physical illnesses.

I told you about the science so you would understand why these strategies are so useful for relieving pain. Pain is like the camel that fell down
under the load of straw. Healing pain is not as simple as removing the
last straw that caused the camel to drop — it was everything else that
was there before, too. You are starting to learn how to get rid of some
of the load that is contributing to your condition. Dr. Alex Cahana has
suggested that "We don't have pain; we do pain."[25] When we change
pain to a verb, we change our relationship to it. There is good reason to
regard pain as something we *do*. We can see from the science discussed
here that mind-body medicine can influence how we perceive pain, that
it can modify our experience — "how we do pain" — and that, most
important, the necessary mind-body skills are teachable.

Now it's your turn. Following are three ways you can start to change
your body chemistry using the science of mind-body medicine, right
now.

Exercise 1

Choose one of the breathing techniques discussed earlier and practice
it every day for a few minutes — while waiting for the bus, for your
computer to boot, or for the kids to get into the car. Start your day with
a breathing exercise, and you may not even need that coffee to wake up.

Exercise 2

Eat one meal each day (or one part of a meal) mindfully. Take a few minutes at every meal to chew your food twice as long as you normally do.

Exercise 3

As you fall asleep at night, bring to your mind the things for which you
are grateful.

CHAPTER 6

HEALTHY HABITS

Nothing so needs reforming as other people's habits.

— Mark Twain

I can think of many good reasons to adopt healthy habits in your daily life. Above all, they will improve your health and your body's ability to heal and will reduce the impact of pain in your life. If you incorporate even a few of these habits, you'll be able to do more of the things you want to do.

Habits are not necessarily voluntary. They can be hardwired into your brain, and when bad habits cause pain, that pain, too, can be hardwired into your brain. Fortunately, making good habits can change the wiring of your brain, which can relieve the pain brought on by bad habits. This is called neuroplasticity, and in chapter 3 I mentioned its potential for treating chronic conditions. Our brains get better at whatever we focus on, just as our bodies get better at sports when we practice. We can train our brains to sharpen our focus on pain or to lessen that focus. Good habits can reduce pain and improve our ability to do the activities that are meaningful to us.

Some habits naturally distract from pain. These distracting habits can be valuable. "Pain is inevitable, suffering is optional," reads a Buddhist proverb. When we are distracted, our pain remains but we reduce our suffering by paying it less attention. For example, one study showed that patients who have a pleasant view from their window after surgery require fewer painkillers. Some other popular forms of distraction are music, movies, puzzles, and books. Other good examples are playing sports, walking in nature, and spending time with friends or lovers. Meditation is a form of conscious distraction that has been shown to reduce both pain and dependence on painkillers.[1]

Our habits can affect our body's chemistry and inflammation. We saw in chapter 4 that inflammation is a response that protects us from infection or irritation. Inflammation can be healing or damaging. When we are healthy, there is a balance between our inflammation and our natural anti-inflammatory system. We have discussed how diet can improve that balance, and in this chapter we will see that healthy habits can do the same.

Quit Smoking

Smoking has been shown to cut life expectancy by ten years.[2] In 1998, smokers in the United States ran up a tab of $167 billion in excess costs for health care and disability. Malcolm Gladwell, in his book *The Tipping Point*, outlines some of the factors that contribute to the smoking habit.[3] Nicotine relieves boredom and stress, it seems to be the domain of sexy and cool people, and heavily addicted smokers are likely to have a genetic predisposition to derive pleasure from nicotine and can tolerate high doses of the poison. Smokers report that cigarettes help relieve their pain, but the downside, including damage to the entire body, greatly outweighs this positive effect.

Quitting smoking is the factor you can control that most significantly reduces your risk of getting a chronic and life-threatening disease. In addition to all the other ways in which smoking damages your health — including causing cancer, emphysema, chronic obstructive pulmonary disease, asthma, and so on — it starves your tissues of oxygen, which makes it difficult for your body to heal. These negative effects often lead to the long-term aggravation of pain conditions.

Cigarette smoke contains chemicals that clog the small blood vessels, called capillaries, that are supposed to keep the spinal bones, called vertebrae, and the cushions between the vertebrae, called discs, healthy. Without a proper blood supply the discs and the vertebrae break down, causing degenerative disc disease. Smokers are three times as likely to develop this disease compared to nonsmokers. In addition, cigarette smokers have poor circulation in general. This hinders the healing of bones — smokers with fractures heal slower and fare far worse with many types of surgery, including orthopedic.

A thermograph is a machine that measures body heat. Body heat comes from blood circulation, and more heat means better circulation. When a thermograph scans a nonsmoker, it shows lots of heat in the center of the body and in the head, and less heat in the arms and legs. Only the tips of a nonsmoker's fingers and toes have almost no heat. If the test is done while a smoker is smoking, the thermograph shows that most of the smoker is lacking heat and circulation, with only a small amount of heat in the brain and around the heart. Poor circulation means restricted blood flow through capillaries,

If I told you I had a drug that could prevent 93 percent of type 2 diabetes, 81 percent of heart attacks, 50 percent of strokes, and 36 percent of all cancers, would you want that drug?

There is no such drug. What if I told you, however, that with a few healthy habits you could achieve those results? Those habits include not smoking; exercising for three and a half hours per week; eating a healthy diet of vegetables, fruits, beans, whole grains, nuts, and seeds, while maintaining a low meat intake; and keeping your body mass index (a measure of body fat) below the obese range.[22]

which prevents oxygen and nutrients from getting to the skin, bones, muscles, and organs. At the same time, the smoker experiences a significant increase in free radical production. Smokers are more prone to a condition called peripheral neuropathy, in which the tiny nerve endings, usually beginning in the hands and feet, are damaged and become painful. Smokers also get more leg ulcers than nonsmokers. Oftentimes these ulcers won't heal, occasionally even leading to gangrene and amputations.

A Good Night's Sleep

Everyone needs it.

Statistics show we are sleeping less, and everything indicates that this is bad for our health. At least 40 percent of Americans report occasional insomnia, and some studies report that the number is as high as 70 percent. Twenty-four percent of us have difficulty sleeping every night or almost every night.[4] There is a higher incidence among women, and the problem gets worse as we age.[5] Although the exact function of sleep is still largely a mystery, some ingenious studies have given us a glimpse into the darkness.

During sleep we have greater heart rate variability. A heart rate of sixty beats per minute does not necessarily mean one beat per second. The interval between two beats may vary greatly from one beat to another. This beat-to-beat variability is a sign of health and a predictor of longevity. A steady one-beat-per-second rhythm usually suggests heart disease or some other serious condition, and it is a predictor of poor health.

Sleep promotes other healthy rhythms as well. When we are sleeping soundly, some of our biological functions line up their rhythms with each other. These functions include our respiratory rate, blood pressure, and brain waves. This same phenomenon happens when we are in a state of meditation, feeling gratitude or appreciation, or "in the zone" that athletes describe when they feel they are functioning at their best.[6] Scientists call this rhythmic synchrony entrainment, and they agree it is good for our health.[7]

Entrainment was first noticed and written about in the seventeenth century by Christian Huygens, a Dutch physicist who invented the pendulum clock. He noticed that if he placed two pendulum clocks next to each other on a wall and swung their pendulums at different rates, they would eventually end up swinging at the same rate. It was ultimately found that the heaviest pendulum pulled the other into its rhythm until they were synchronized.

Melatonin, a hormone secreted by the pineal gland in our brain when we are in darkness, entrains our body rhythms with the day–night cycle. It is a powerful antioxidant, helps in modulating our immune system, and may discourage the growth of certain cancer cells. Proper melatonin levels affect sexual development and quality of sleep and overall play a role in slowing down the aging processes.[8] The amount of melatonin released from the pineal gland is proportionate to the length of night. In this way, melatonin gives other body systems information about the time of day and time of year. Studies have shown that when we sleep in total darkness, we secrete more melatonin. Even a small amount of light hitting our closed eyelids drastically reduces the amount of melatonin released into our bodies. Only red light does not have this effect. When we sleep with light from a nightlight or even a crack through the window shades, our melatonin secretion plummets. Sadly, these days it can be hard to find a night's sleep in total darkness; a picture taken from space of the modern world at night shows a sea of bright lights.

In addition to getting too much light exposure at night, most of us who live in industrialized countries do not get enough exposure to the right kind of light during the day. We are exposed to artificial light rather than the full spectrum of natural light. This has been shown to cause

SLEEP APNEA

People with sleep apnea stop breathing during their sleep. This can increase the risk of heart attack and stroke, and it can cause high blood pressure, daytime sleepiness, and more. If you snore loudly, gasp for air in the night, or feel unrested upon waking, you may need a sleep test.

seasonal affective disorder, a form of depression more common in the winter months. A robust secretion of melatonin depends on exposure both to natural light during the day and to darkness at night — the conditions of human life at its beginnings in the peri-equatorial African-Syrian Rift Valley. Our lifestyles may have changed, but for the most part our genetics have not. At times, our modern life puts us out of sync with some of the needs of our biological systems.

During sleep we recover from the activities of wakefulness. Our bodies rebuild stores of molecules by replacing or repairing damaged molecules needed for the next day. When we are deprived of sleep, the brain makes molecules that are ordinarily associated with stress — proteins that don't fold properly and that clump together, and heat-shock proteins that are designed to help the body cope with stress. So if you sleep well, you have a tune-up overnight; and if you don't sleep well, your system experiences cellular stress.[9] Sleep also reduces inflammation and improves immune function. There has been speculation about other "off-line" functions performed by the brain during sleep, such as keeping memory tuned up and fit by exercising it with dreams, and refreshing circuits for new memories. Consequently, sleep is restorative, and a lack of sleep is associated with fatigue and cognitive impairment.

Research has shown that people who don't sleep well, who work night shifts, or who have jet lag can develop health problems at a higher rate than those with regular sleep patterns. People also have difficulty losing weight if they are not sleeping well.

The conventional wisdom is that we need seven or eight hours of sleep per night. Research shows that people who live in industrialized

Once, when I was in medical school, I went to bed preoccupied with a difficult exam question. At some point in the night, I got up and scribbled something on a piece of paper in the dark. When I woke up in the morning, I remembered the incident but not what I had written. I was surprised to discover that my nocturnal note was not gibberish, as I had expected, but the correct solution to the problem!

countries and get this much sleep are healthier than those who get less. We should wake up feeling refreshed and have no daytime drowsiness.

Here are some habits that can help you get a good night's sleep. Adopt a regular sleep time and develop a relaxing bedtime routine. During the hour or two before bed, do not consume large quantities of food or beverages, exercise vigorously, or focus on aggravating issues. In addition, avoid using a computer or watching TV; the light from computer screens and TVs excites the brain. Keep your bedroom cool, dark, and quiet. Go to bed tired and turn out the lights. Have a comfortable mattress and pillow. Sleep primarily at night, and limit daytime naps to a maximum of thirty minutes. Sleep in total darkness or use a sleep mask. Avoid nicotine, and limit nighttime caffeine, alcohol, and sugar consumption. All of these chemicals are stimulants. Nicotine is an outright stimulant, as is caffeine. Alcohol makes you drowsy at first, but then wakes you up a few hours later. Some people are more sensitive to these chemicals; and if you have any trouble sleeping, completely avoid them to reestablish a healthy sleep pattern.

ENTRAINING A CHILD TO SLEEP

One of my children never liked to go to sleep. He was wakeful from his earliest moments. Once he was out of his crib (he climbed out at nine months and slept on a mattress on the floor after that), I got into a routine of lying down beside him and putting him to sleep with a breathing exercise. I would match my breathing rate to his and slowly lengthen my breaths. Without knowing what was happening, he would alter his breathing pattern to match mine — it would become entrained — and soon he would be asleep. When he was about two years old, he figured out that I was doing something that made him tired almost against his will. One day as I lay down beside him, he said, "Don't do whatever you do that makes me fall asleep."

As we age, we tend to sleep less at night and take daytime naps. We don't really understand all the reasons for this, but there may be some practical causes, such as needing to get up to pee.

There is some interesting research on sleep that suggests interrupted sleep is not the big problem. In fact, it seems worrying about interrupted sleep is the real problem. Professor A. Roger Ekirch, who teaches history at Virginia Polytechnic Institute and State University, researched the sleep patterns of humans during preindustrial times, before we had artificial lights.[10] He found that interrupted nighttime sleep was considered normal, and that people at the time thought of sleep as being composed of two segments — "first sleep" and "second sleep." In between the two segments, people would stay awake for several hours, using the time to think about their day, do chores, or even go visiting. Sleep was preceded by what sleep specialists call a long latency, meaning it took a long time to fall asleep. In modern times, we might call this a sleep disorder, but perhaps it is the natural human pattern, needed to quiet the brain and transition it to an alternate state of consciousness. Thomas A. Wehr, MD, professor emeritus at the National Institute of Mental Health, studied this phenomenon and questions whether our modern sleep patterns are unnatural and cause chronic sleep deprivation.[11] Perhaps many of the "sleep disorders" that find their way into doctors' offices and generate endless prescriptions for sleep medications are just natural sleep patterns.

It is important to find a comfortable sleeping position for the neck, back, arms, and legs. A pillow that provides neck support is crucial. If you sleep on your side, make certain the pillow comes right down to support the entire length of your neck. Your neck is like a suspension bridge, and if your pillow supports only your head, then your neck muscles are left unsupported and unable to rest. Whether you sleep on your side or back, a pillow that has a ridge along the lower edge is useful because it will conform to the contours of your neck. There are so many neck pillows on the market that it can be difficult to decide on one without trying them out. This can get expensive, so I recommend you experiment by rolling up a towel and placing it inside your pillow case, at the bottom of your pillow. See if you can determine the size and firmness of the contour that works for you. Adjustable pillows, such as buckwheat or water pillows, are useful. Buckwheat pillows can be warmed in the microwave. If you tend not to move around a lot at night, a small, soft pillow bunched up under your neck may be all you need.

SILK BEDDING

My personal bedding favorites are silk-filled duvets and pillows, both covered in 100 percent cotton. These will keep you warm but won't overheat you. They also repel dust mites and don't create the static electricity that synthetics and other fibers do.

If you are a side sleeper, you can place a large body pillow in front of you to support your top arm. This is helpful for shoulder and arm pain and will also keep you from rolling over. You might also find it comfortable to have a pillow behind you, to keep yourself from tossing around at night. If you sleep on your side, you should also try lying with your bottom arm out behind you instead of in front. If you sleep on your back, you may find that a pillow under your knees helps your low back. This is a good position that encourages your pectoral muscles to relax and allows your shoulder blades to slide toward the spine. If you have neck and shoulder problems, you might benefit from sleeping on a slight incline with your head and shoulders elevated. You can purchase foam wedges for this purpose. As an added bonus, sleeping on your back, according to the American Academy of Dermatology, helps to reduce facial wrinkles.

If you sleep on your stomach, you might consider breaking the habit — it strains your neck. If you must sleep in this position, try wedging a large body pillow under one side of your torso. With a pillow there, you will be lying on an angle, not fully on your stomach, and your neck will be in a more neutral position.

In his book on sleep, *Healing Night*, Rubin R. Naiman, PhD, discusses the importance of dreams to a good night's sleep.[12] He believes that dreaming, which he calls psychological stretching, is essential to our well-being. Dreams are as important as sleep, but most sleep medications on the market suppress the dream phase of sleep. These medications should be used with caution, not only because of their effect on dreams, but also because most of them are highly addictive.

Dental Care

When you want to know how healthy a horse is, you look in its mouth. Teeth and gum health is very important to the overall health of humans as well. For example, gum inflammation called gingivitis is not only a dental problem but also a catalyst for disease in general; inflamed gums provide an entry site for many infections.

With modern dental practices and good daily self-care, we can expect to keep our own teeth for a lifetime. Regular brushing and flossing are essential to dental health, as is a proper diet and regular checkups.

WHAT DOCTORS LEARN ABOUT DENTISTRY

We learned little about dental diseases and dental care in medical school. I recently reviewed the medical "bible" *Harrison's Principles of Medicine* from my medical school days, and I noticed that in more than two thousand pages, dental health gets only a couple of columns. Needless to say, the book says little about the connection between dental and overall health.

Be aware, though, that not all of modern dental care is safe, and I recommend avoiding some substances. Many countries have already banned the use of amalgam fillings containing mercury.[13] The World Health Organization's position in 2005 on the use of mercury was clear: they supported "a ban for use of mercury containing devices and effectively promote the use of mercury free alternatives."[14] Mercury is a known neurotoxin, and viable alternatives called resins are available. Some white resins used for dental work, however, contain bisphenol A, a harmful additive used in manufacturing plastics. It has been banned from use in baby bottles in Canada, and exposure limits have been set in Europe. When toxins are present in your dental work, you experience long-term, low-dose exposure. This type of exposure is difficult to research. There is also a growing controversy over fluoride, and it seems that there is growing support for banning it from drinking water. The benefits of fluoride were never clearly proven, and there may be toxicity associated with it.

There are dentists who practice "biological dentistry," who have mercury-free offices and steer clear of harmful resins and fluoride.

Prepare for the Weather

We have lost touch with our environment in so many ways. One indicator for me was my children, who when they were little hated dressing for the weather. They grew up living in the Northeast, where we had harsh winters and hot, muggy summers. As soon as they were too old for me to choose their outfits, they began opening up their jackets in winter, their hats stayed on the hall tree, and their gloves disappeared entirely. I think maybe one of them wore boots. I remember lecturing them on the importance of protecting themselves from the elements. "You never know," I urged them. "If your bus or car breaks down, you might have to walk five miles through a blizzard and subzero temperatures to safety!" They laughed at me. If I was lucky, they would stuff a hat in a pocket before going on their way.

We lived in a large urban center. They were right, in a way: they couldn't have walked a block without running into several options for shelter. But the principle is still a good one, especially for people in pain: respect nature and the elements.

In winter, and in air-conditioned spaces during other seasons, it is important to keep your body from getting chilled. Too much cold causes your blood vessels to constrict and your muscles to tighten. This hinders blood circulation and may increase pain. Additionally, any sudden drop in body temperature causes a stress reaction, which can increase pain and your vulnerability to infection.

In summer, it is important to hydrate. Dehydration happens when your body uses more water than it consumes, and it is very easy to be dehydrated in hot, dry weather — you sweat more, and sometimes it can be hard to tell you are sweating. If you don't urinate at least five times a day, you should be drinking more water. In addition, your urine should

HUNGER OR THIRST?

Sometimes when you feel hungry, you're actually in need of water and not food. If hunger strikes when you aren't due for a regular meal, try a glass of water instead. If that satisfies you, then you've saved yourself some unnecessary calories.

be a pale yellow. A headache and tiredness are early signs of dehydration. Get in the habit of drinking when you're thirsty. Of course, drinking is not the only way to hydrate. Fruits and vegetables too contain plenty of water.

Sunburns are harmful. They cause cancer, premature aging of the skin, and suppression of the immune system. Nevertheless, sunlight in general is not dangerous — it has nurtured life on earth for billions of years. Many of my pain patients find relief in the sun, and limited periods of exposure without sunscreen, around twenty minutes' worth each day, are healthy for most of us. Those with a family history of melanoma, the most serious form of skin cancer, are the exception. These individuals should avoid the sun until further research determines if there is a safe level of sun exposure for people with family histories of melanoma.

Sunscreens are controversial. While they prevent redness of the skin from sun exposure, they probably don't prevent cancer. Sunscreen sales are at a record high, and cases of melanoma are not decreasing — in fact, they are rising steadily. Research is currently being done on the different components of sunscreen and how they react with one another when heated on our skin. Some of these components may be toxic and may actually cause cancer. To avoid lengthy sun exposure, find shade or cover up with clothing. Save sunscreens for times when long periods of sun exposure are absolutely unavoidable.

Vitamin D deficiency is common in the Northern Hemisphere. In the summer, a little sun exposure will make your skin produce its own vitamin D. This is not the case, however, during winter in the Northern Hemisphere.

Sun exposure may also tune up our immune system through the exposure of our immune and blood cells to light, through our skin.

Making Use of Heat and Cold

Both cold and heat can relieve pain. General wisdom has always suggested that, following an injury, ice should be used for the first twenty-four to forty-eight hours, after which heat is better. I find this works, but there are some people who prefer cold for even long-standing pain. Other chronic pain sufferers cannot stand any cold applications, while others still cannot stand cold applications but still appreciate liniments that give the sensation of cold, such as menthol. Menthol temporarily reduces blood flow in the skin by causing vasoconstriction, which may actually block some of the natural chemicals that cause pain.

Heat increases blood flow by causing local vasodilation — the expansion of blood vessels. At times, this makes swelling worse. Although cold reduces blood flow when applied, it can cause vasodilation when removed.

People in pain often experience cold hands and feet. For cold extremities, Janet Travell recommends applying heat to the abdomen. Once the core of the body is heated, she explains, the extremities draw the heat away from the core. In this way, all the extremities warm simultaneously.[15]

A far-infrared sauna is a useful form of heating for many reasons. This type of sauna is unlike other saunas because the air in it is dry and warm, but not hot, so breathing is easy and you can stay in it comfortably for thirty minutes or longer. In it, your body is heated through infrared light, which penetrates through your skin and into deeper structures. It improves circulation and helps detoxify your body by causing toxins such as heavy metals and modern chemicals to come out in your sweat. It has been shown to improve the healing of injuries and is used by athletes for this purpose.

People with fibromyalgia often feel relief in a far-infrared sauna. Typically, postmenopausal women do not like excess heat, but they often like this type of sauna. (Caution: pregnant women and people with certain diseases, such as myasthenia gravis, should not overheat their bodies.)

Work

Work is highly important to North Americans. Many people tie their self-image to their work and spend far more than half of their waking hours doing it. Some individuals find so much satisfaction in their work that they get sick as soon as they retire. Our work can take on a rhythm that seems unstoppable, and many times illness is a wake-up call for those who work too hard. In these cases, even serious illness can be seen as a blessing that allows us to rebalance our priorities. It's healthy to think of work as more than just "making a living," and work can be a good distraction for pain patients. Nevertheless, balancing work with social and family life is also important for our health.

Work is specifically important for those with pain problems. When I codirected a clinic for people with work-related, repetitive strain injuries in Toronto, we tried to keep our pain patients at work even if it was their work activities that had injured them. Over 90 percent of our patients stayed at work, many of them with workplace modifications. Their improvements in therapy were a little slower, because they were still doing the injuring activities, but most of them felt that the overall outcome was better. If you have a pain problem and it's at all reasonable for you to stay at work, you should. Continuing your work will keep you conditioned for work activities, and you will avoid the long reintroduction to work once your injury improves. Additionally, your work will give you something to focus on besides your pain.

People in pain often live their lives focusing on their pain. As I mentioned earlier, neuroplasticity means that this focus can rewire the brain to favor pain messages — making them stronger and able to move faster. One way for pain patients to avoid this is to keep involved in as many activities as possible, and staying at work is one option. If you absolutely can't stay at work, find a charity to volunteer for, in whatever capacity you can. Serving a meal at a homeless shelter, or volunteering with the elderly or with children, can give you satisfaction and make you feel useful, which will keep you healthy and reduce your pain.

Make a Home

You should think of your home as a safe, relaxing place where you can go to rest and recover from a day's activities. You don't need a lot of money to make your home beautiful. Give some thought to what you like to look at, have music available, and try to get some good lighting. Some of us live in climates where there is little natural light for much of the year. There are full-spectrum lightbulbs that will give you more exposure to natural light. During the winter, these bulbs can curb grumpy moods that come from a lack of natural light.

Family, Friends, Self

In the olden days, people lived their whole lives in the same town, city, or region. They were connected to their land, relatives, and neighbors. Travel was expensive, slow, and sometimes dangerous. A few adventurous souls explored faraway places, but the majority of people were laid to rest in the same cemeteries as their grandparents. In those days, family and community held more significance. Family was a place you could go if you had nowhere else — where you always felt you belonged. And those in a community looked out for each other.

Inexpensive, high-speed travel and communication have changed our world for the better...and perhaps also for the worse. In our new, global village, we are constantly connected to everyone; our family and friends are never more than a click or a plane ticket away. Nevertheless, many people find themselves alone, in exciting circumstances but disconnected from their families and communities — their "tribe." In our global village, it's not always easy to find a hug or someone to feel close to. Family and community are easily taken for granted and their roles diminished.

Practicing random acts of kindness and feeling gratitude are associated with positive emotions.

In times of trouble, it is natural to yearn for connection to those who know you and accept you. According to shamanic tradition and aboriginal cultures, these connections extend beyond family to community. Illness is seen as a community problem, and the solution also involves community. These days, the lack of meaningful social connection and the separation from traditions and rituals leave many people struggling to maintain equilibrium when they hit life's storms. Many are so estranged from their roots that they hardly know what they have lost. They may have a sense of disconnection that is profound and lasts a lifetime.

But caring connections have been shown over and over to enhance health, prolong life, and offer most of us our most meaningful moments. Cardiologist, researcher, and author Dean Ornish is famous for showing us that a low-fat diet can improve heart health. He also points out that connection, affection, and love in our lives are even more important than diet and give us the greatest survival benefits. Love and connection to family and community help people survive difficult times. UCLA's Shelley Taylor, PhD, has studied human connections and their impact on health. She describes how oxytocin, a hormone whose level jumps when we are stressed, makes us reach out for caring relationships — something she calls the "tend and befriend" response.[16] Physical contact like touching and hugging between family, friends, or lovers increases the levels of calming oxytocin, which in turn lowers stress-hormone levels. Oxytocin is important in mother-infant bonding and has other health benefits, such as decreasing heart disease and increasing lifespan in cancer patients. Oxytocin is anti-inflammatory.

Oftentimes, when those in the hospital cry, whether old or young, they cry out for their first connection, their mothers. Their mothers may not be close by, or even alive, but that first human connection can still have profound impact if only through the memory of their caring presence. In our fast-paced lives, sometimes we forget to nurture our connections with family and friends. We think we have things to do that are more important than the gifts we simultaneously give and receive when we reach out to those who care about us. We should make it a habit to connect.

In many instances, however, people's early connections were destructive and abusive. For people who have had such difficult relationships in the past, learning to trust others requires work using appropriate psychological healing techniques. Those who have experienced an abusive or traumatic past are more likely to develop chronic pain conditions.

Self-care is important too. As the saying goes, if we don't know how to love ourselves, then we also don't know how to love others. The scholar Hillel, who lived about two thousand years ago, wrote, "If I am not for myself, who will be for me? But if I am only for myself, what am I? And if not now, when?" When it comes to relationships, we need to balance our inward focus with our outward focus. We need to know how to care for ourselves, determine our needs, and balance them with the needs of the significant people in our lives. This entire chapter is about self-care.

I speak with many people who don't think they have the time to look after themselves, because they are too busy looking after everyone else at home, at work, and at play. At times in my life, I myself have been guilty of that. Eventually, however, I realized that I would not be able to look after anyone else if I didn't take time to follow my own advice and take care of myself. Caring for myself has been one of the most difficult lessons for me to learn, and my children, the recipients of much of my caring, have been instrumental in my learning it. They saw my health deteriorate and got angry with me for giving good advice to others and not following it myself. Thank you, my sweet children, for calling me out for my hypocrisy.

Play

There are countless ways to "play." You could play an instrument, play a sport, play a computer game, or go to a theatrical play where "players" play others. To play is to be "not serious," to be outside the boundaries of ordinary life, to be lighthearted. Although there are psychology books devoted to the definitions of play and its benefits, it is still difficult to define — yet we all know what it is. One of the most-quoted books about play is aptly called *The Ambiguity of Play*.[17] Nevertheless, everyone agrees that play is important for all ages. During play we integrate the left, analytical, side of our brain with the right, creative, side. Make sure to take time out of your schedule, no matter how busy, and play. Play wholeheartedly, as you did when you were a child. Lose yourself in the joy of it.

The Senses and Sensuality

Treat your body with loving-kindness. All of it — even the part that hurts. It is after all still a part of you and not apart from you. Yet pain sufferers sometimes have a difficult time feeling love for the part that hurts and sometimes even reject it.

I don't think it helps to treat your painful part as something foreign to your body. If your brain focuses too much on that thought, it may have difficulty reintegrating the painful part as you heal. Some patients with a condition called chronic regional pain syndrome severely reject an injured and painful part, and even ask to have it amputated. Unfortunately, amputation does not improve the pain and may even add to it. Evidence suggests that in all cases of pain, including chronic regional pain syndrome, it helps to treat your painful body part as normally as possible. Move it as normally as you can and think of and care for it with kindness.

When you're in pain, you might find it hard to focus on anything else. You may occupy your whole self with the part that hurts. This is a natural instinct and with acute pain, it might be a matter of survival. For example, if your hand is on the stove, it's very important that you stop everything you're doing and attend to it. Chronic pain, however, is different, and focusing on that pain is probably not necessary for survival.

Attention to your senses can be a path to pain relief. This includes all of the senses: touch, smell, taste, sight, and hearing. Try allowing any of your senses to be your focus at any given moment. Not only is this a meditative practice that can distract you from your pain, but it can also change your brain and body chemistry, which can give chemical pain relief. Try spending time looking at nature, eating a favorite food slowly, or going for a massage. These different sensations are ways of shifting your focus away from pain and onto something that is associated with pleasure.

Some people in pain have decreased interest in sex. This may be caused by the pain itself or by the side effects of medications, mostly anti-depressants or opioids. Nevertheless, sex can promote pain relief. Creativity may be needed to accommodate different activities and positions that are comfortable for the partner in pain. Sometimes a couple will need to be more focused on sharing pleasure together and not on a specific outcome. For some pain patients, sex gives hours of pain relief, perhaps because it releases endorphins, but also perhaps because it reawakens the sense of connection and the joy of living.

Music and Art

Music is energy. We are made up of cells, which are made up of molecules and atoms, all of which have vibrating energies. So it makes sense that music should affect us at a cellular level.

Music has touched my life. When I was little, my mother used to take me to Massey Hall in Toronto — a darkly lit concert hall with steep balconies and wooden fold-up seats. We would go to listen to the Kiwanis Festival finalists. In high school, my sister and her friends went to concerts at student rates, and I followed their lead and organized a group of friends to attend a series of concerts. I loved those concerts. I liked the black-and-white concert attire, the concentrated faces of the musicians, and the gyrations of the conductor, a dynamic and then very young Seiji Ozawa. How wonderful it was that society paid people to follow a career to bring us music!

I always loved to sing, but, conscious of my inability to carry a tune, I usually confined my arias to the shower or the car with the windows rolled up, and I sang to my children, who, bless them, accepted my voice for the love it carried. Music was always around our home. My husband played piano for sing-alongs, I took my children to music classes, and we would sing at bedtimes. There was a lull in music when my kids were at the age when they attended activities that required parents to act as chauffeurs. And there was a particularly difficult time in my life when I found I could not listen to music without crying — music brings you closer to your emotions. During that period, I avoided music because the hectic pace of my life had to continue; I had no time to cry, so I had no time for music and the emotions it brought out in me.

As my children grew up, they began to discover the music of the fifties, sixties, and seventies that I had known. I was able to reconnect to the tunes and rhythms that had permeated my youth. I started to listen to all kinds of music again.

A few years ago, after moving to Arizona, I got ill with valley fever. During that time, I went through months when my body was wracked with pain. Just getting out of bed in the morning seemed more than I was capable of. Pain and restlessness would not allow me to sleep. My wonderful friend Carrie shared with me the meditation music written for the healer Bruno Groening. This finally motivated me to learn to use one of the iPods that my kids were so attached to. I would listen to what I called "Bruno music" and fall into restful sleep, my agitation and pain relieved for hours. I found I could get up in the morning for a few hours after listening to it again. This music became my healing companion and saw me through a very difficult time.

In his book *The Healing Power of Sound*, Mitchell Gaynor outlines his own journey into the connection between the vibrational energy of sound and its impact on the human body. He uses it extensively as a means of connecting cancer patients with their truest selves and opening pathways to optimism, pain relief, and healing. Up to now, I have used very little music in my medical practice. While writing this book, however, I have become more aware of its potential healing benefits, and I will certainly apply that awareness to my future practice.

Connection with beauty in life is good for the soul. For the most part, music and art connect, rather than divide, people. Beauty exists in many unlikely places, as photographers show us in their photos of nature and people, and even of graffiti, slums, and urban decay. Many of us have never explored our creativity. We don't have to be extremely talented or professionals to make our creativity worthwhile. The activity of creating something, not the end product, is the important part. Good creative activities include knitting, needlework, painting, drawing, making pottery, stringing beads, sculpting, whittling wood, taking photos, and putting other people's photos into collages. Deepak Chopra, MD, a well-known holistic healer and author, said, "Experiencing gratitude is one of the most effective ways of getting in touch with your soul."[18] It is easy to be grateful for the beauty of art, whether it was created by ourselves or others.

Animals

My father was a gentle man who taught me many important life lessons. Among those lessons was a love for children and animals. Children and animals live in the present with authenticity. They can also sense the energy and emotion in a situation. They read beyond the superficial words and niceties that punctuate many interactions in the "adult" world.

Research has shown that petting a dog can lower your blood pressure. Dogs can calm anxieties and provide unconditional affection, which is rare in our lives. When your dog greets you at the front door, it cares little if you messed up at work, forgot to pick up the dry cleaning, or flunked a test. If you take the time and relate to that affection, it will help you shed the stresses of the day. This will change your body's chemistry for the better.

Most cats have a different way of relating to their keepers. Despite their independent nature, however, they still confer a calming effect and health benefits on their owners. The authors of one study noticed that fractures in cats heal more quickly than fractures in dogs. It turns out that the vibrational frequency of a cat's purr helps heal broken bones and relieves pain.

Horses have an astonishing connection with humans. If they have not been mistreated by humans, they are mostly gentle, sweet animals with good hearts. They are also prey animals and sense the emotions of those around them. They keep you honest. Horses are used in therapeutic settings for these very reasons. They help people become more authentic with their emotions. When you experience your true emotion, the body language of the horse changes and it becomes relaxed. This helps you and your therapist discover how you really feel about things. Horses running and grazing in a field are one of the most beautiful sights. It brings me the same feeling of awe and peace as does seeing an eagle soar, a maritime sunset, or majestic mountains. I know many pain patients who are horseback riders and experience relief while riding.

For many years I have had animals in my life. Caring for them becomes part of a nurturing, daily ritual. I still think fondly of the eight months I looked after my daughter's horse in our little barn in the backyard in Tucson. As I would walk down the long lane from the house, I could see the horse strain her neck upward to see me. She welcomed me with a whinny and a nuzzle. I feel happy just thinking about it.

Happiness

We who lived in concentration camps can remember the men who walked through the huts comforting others, giving away their last piece of bread. They may have been few in number, but they offer sufficient proof that everything can be taken from a man but one thing: the last of the human freedoms — to choose one's attitude in any given set of circumstances, to choose one's own way.

— VIKTOR FRANKL, *Man's Search for Meaning*

Happiness is a habit. It is also a choice you can make every day. You can focus on every annoying detail that comes your way, or you can choose to be happy. We all know people who are inexplicably happy even when they face serious difficulties in their lives. We also know others who can find fault with even the most perfect moment. There are many things in our lives that we do not have control over, but we do have control over our reactions and our attitudes.

There are factors of nature and nurture that affect how we respond to events in our lives.[19] Some people instinctively look at the positive side of each situation. They find the joyful spot in life even when most of what is happening is difficult or tragic. They can still feel joy at the sunrise, smile when they see a friend or child, or feel comfort at simply recalling a past, sweet memory. Martin Seligman developed a field of psychology called positive psychology.[20] He says it involves five elements — positive emotion; engagement with or concentrated attention to whatever you are doing at the moment; relationships; meaning and purpose, or being involved in something that is bigger than the self; and accomplishment. It turns out that there are clear health advantages to positive psychology. In one study of nuns, the happiest people in the study were four times more likely to live to old age as the least happy people.[21] In addition, the happy nuns did not develop dementia symptoms, while the less happy sisters did.

Optimism is closely tied to happiness. According to Merriam-Webster's, fifteenth edition, optimism is "an inclination to put the most favorable construction upon actions and events or to anticipate the best possible outcome." This definition ties optimism to a positive outcome. I like the definition of optimism as the belief that things will be fine even if you don't get the perfect outcome. This is more in line with Gottfried Wilhelm Leibniz, a seventeenth-century philosopher who described optimism as simply the attitude that this world is the best of all possible worlds.

Being happy and optimistic is not about ignoring the negative emotions. It is important to recognize the entire range of our emotions — positive and negative. We can be aware of our sadness, irritation, anger, frustration, jealousy, and grief without letting them dominate our lives. Awareness of these emotions helps us calm ourselves, manage our emotions, practice being a good listener, practice empathy, and give constructive feedback.

As I mentioned earlier, positivity is affected by nature and nurture. While some people are

HAPPINESS AS A HABIT

"Authentic happiness comes from identifying and cultivating your most fundamental strengths and using them every day in work, love, play and parenting."
– Martin Seligman,
Authentic Happiness

born with a more positive outlook, you can also develop your positive side by practicing. These are learnable skills.

Meaning in Life

Abby is a fifty-five-year-old woman who spent her life working hard. She is tall and slim and has muscular arms. She worked in construction her entire life and is proud that she could do heavy work just like the men did. She is a Native American whose parents, brothers, and sisters still live on the reservation, but she and her husband moved to a city with their children to find work. Her husband died several years ago. All her children are grown now, and she lives with one of her daughters, her son-in-law, and their children. A while ago, she developed some stomach symptoms, and the doctors were not certain of the cause. She had her gallbladder removed because her doctors thought it might help. It didn't. Next, she had a rarely done surgery to tighten the muscles at the top of the stomach because her doctors thought her problem might be heartburn (GERD). That didn't help, either. Instead, the two consecutive surgeries caused a weakness in the muscles of her abdomen, and she developed pain in her abdomen and her right side. When she tried to lift anything or bend over, she would feel her stomach bulging out through the weak muscles. Her doctors tried to reinforce the muscles by reoperating and putting in a piece of synthetic mesh. The pain got worse. She got physical therapy to help her strengthen her muscles, but nothing changed. After a while, the surgeon decided that the mesh might be causing some of her problems and removed it, saying there was nothing more that could be done.

"Act as if what you do makes a difference. It does."
– William James

When Abby comes to see me, I start her on acupuncture and cold laser treatments. These treatments gradually give her some relief and help her get through the day with less pain. She is on opioids, sedatives, and two antidepressants. She is sad over her losses, but not really depressed. I suggest she slowly wean herself off one of the antidepressants to see if it has actually been helping her. After a few more months, she stops taking all of her drugs except for the opioids, and she begins weaning herself off those too. She is deficient in vitamin D, and she starts taking high doses. I also convince her to eat more vegetables and give up soda. She really wants to go back to work and tries to help at a drywall job. She had been so proud of her work, and it had given her life additional meaning. Without it, she feels useless. After a serious talk with me, she realizes she may never be able to do that work again. This greatly distresses her.

Whenever Abby is in my office, I notice that she doodles on the questionnaire forms. Her sketches are detailed and beautiful. I begin to speak to her about her art, and she dismisses it as unimportant. At subsequent visits, however, she tells me that on construction jobs, she was the one who would add artistic details to the project. She never thought of those details as important. Over the next two months, Abby shifts her thinking and begins to regard herself as an artist. Now, she paints and is planning an exhibit where her parents live. She still has pain in her stomach and back at times, but she has learned to manage it with some exercises, mind-body techniques, and drugs when she needs them. She tells me the biggest difference is that pain does not run her life anymore. Having found new meaning in life, she has become more than just her pain.

CHAPTER 7

DIETARY SUPPLEMENTS

*We believe a daily multivitamin-multimineral pill offers safe,
simple micronutrient insurance.*

— HARVARD SCHOOL OF PUBLIC HEALTH,
"Nutrition Insurance Policy: A Daily Multivitamin"

Shahira is a forty-seven-year-old administrative assistant. She is overweight and has been told she is prediabetic. She used to be active, swimming and playing tennis in her twenties and thirties. In her forties, however, she has found that raising her children, caring for her ailing elderly parents, helping her husband with his business ventures, and maintaining her status at work have left no time for sports. She has early arthritis in both knees and, at times, walks with a limp owing to hip pain. She has been to her family doctor repeatedly, who first told her to take acetaminophen and later to switch to an over-the-counter anti-inflammatory. She eats a diet based on the food pyramid and drinks diet soda. She wonders why she keeps gaining weight. She feels tired and does not sleep well. Her knees are now too sore for exercise, and she feels she is on an inevitable path toward knee replacement surgery and ill health. She takes four acetaminophen and two anti-inflammatories every day just to get through the day. Her stomach hurts from the drugs. Her doctor gives her a stronger anti-inflammatory and a drug to protect her stomach. He also suggests an antidepressant and another pill for sleep. Shahira looks at all the pill bottles. She does not like the idea of taking so many foreign chemicals, and she is worried about her future health.

Fortunately for Shahira, she develops some wrist pain at work that is mistakenly diagnosed as carpal tunnel syndrome, and she is referred to a clinic specializing in the treatment of work-related disorders. This is a clinic that practices integrative medicine, and when Shahira gets there she has a full assessment. In telling her own story of the stresses in her life, it becomes clear to Shahira that she feels she is buckling under a burden. She explores with the doctor how she is neglecting her own health. She listens carefully to the suggestions of this doctor and decides to take his advice. After caring for so many others in her life, she now needs to pay attention to herself — to her own health. She is heartened when the doctor tells her that she can improve her health in all the areas she is concerned about, not just the numbness and pain in her hands.

For homework, Shahira is told to buy a book on low-glycemic eating and to begin planning all her food intake according to those guidelines. She learns about the research on pain and omega-3 fish oils, B vitamins, magnesium, and vitamin D. She discusses with the doctor the doses of these she should take. She learns about the importance of eating many vegetables every day. She learns about the importance of restorative sleep. She had been giving herself only five to six hours of sleep at night and spent much of that time tossing and turning owing to stress and discomfort. Since her knees are too painful for her to walk for her exercise, the doctor suggests that Shahira try exercising in water three times a week for at least half an hour. He also refers her to a physical therapist to learn specific exercises, and to a massage therapist to get treatments for the painful knots in her muscles.

Shahira goes home and tells her husband all she has learned. She explains to her parents and her grown children that she now needs some time to look after herself. After all, if she becomes disabled, she won't be able to help them, either.

Six weeks later, she returns to the doctor to report on her progress. She has been taking B vitamins, vitamin D, and fish oils and has just started taking magnesium. She also has worked with the physical and massage therapists and even made time to get to the pool a few times. She is amazed at how well she feels. Her wrist, knee, and hip pain is reduced. She sleeps eight hours a night, and soundly. She hadn't realized that the side effects of her supplements would be improved sleep and improved coping skills for stress. She feels hopeful that she can improve her health overall and is pleased with the results of her low-glycemic eating. Her husband has changed his diet as well, and they both notice that their clothes are looser — especially around the waist.

Now that Shahira understands she can control her health problems through nutrition and lifestyle, she wants more information about how to continue on this path to healing. She wants to stop the over-the-counter painkillers. The doctor tells her about some other things that can help, including ginger, turmeric, and quercetin.

Dietary supplements, or nutritional supplements, are vitamins, minerals, and other nutrients, usually taken as pills. They can also be medicinal plants and their extracts. The vitamins, magnesium, and fish oil that Shahira takes are supplements. So are the ginger, turmeric, and quercetin.

Every day, your body suffers countless injuries. Most of the time, these injuries are tiny and healthful ones, and your body quickly heals them. For example, when you work out, you make tiny tears in your muscles; your body then rebuilds those muscles bigger and stronger. This rebuilding is healing, and it requires raw

NOTE TO READERS

If you are considering supplements be sure to consult with your health care provider to ensure you are taking the proper doses of the proper supplements. Some supplements may not be recommended for certain individuals, depending on their health.[1]

VITAMIN STUDIES NEED SPECIAL METHODS

More research is needed on the association of health outcomes and vitamin use. Often the research done tries to use individual nutrients as though they are drugs. The effects of drugs tend to be dramatic, happen over a short period of time, and can be accompanied by side effects: the risk of significant disruptions of the body's natural systems. Nutrients work synergistically with one another and are not "new-to-nature" molecules like drugs are.

materials. Healing works best when your body has the materials it is preprogrammed to use, which means nutrients — food and dietary supplements. This is why, when promoting healing and treating pain, food and supplements are my first line of therapy. Food is always best, but supplements are close behind.

Major universities have supplied excellent research on nutritional supplements, and I cite some in the footnotes. Although some products listed here need further, more extensive study, I believe they are worth trying, especially since they have such a low risk of causing harm. Many also have plausible mechanisms of action — that is, there's a plausible explanation for how they work — and a long history of successful use in traditional medical systems such as Ayurveda, Traditional Chinese Medicine, and aboriginal healing practices. The same nutrients affect all systems of the body, so supplements do have side effects. The good news is that these side effects are almost always beneficial.

Dose and Quality

When taking supplements, finding a dose appropriate to you can be a bit confusing, and there are two official guides you should be aware of — the recommended daily allowance (RDA) and the "tolerable upper intake level."

The RDA often does not take into account how much of a nutrient is needed for optimal health, and more research is needed in this area. The RDA often defines minimum levels, which are sometimes not even adequate to prevent disease — a subject I discuss in the section on vitamin D. Research by Roger Williams, PhD, a highly respected University of Texas professor, shows we all need different amounts of the specific nutrients, based on our unique characteristics.[2] His research also shows that our needs can change from day to day, depending on stress. Recommended daily allowances also do not take into account this individual or day-to-day variability in nutrient requirements.

The "tolerable upper intake level" is another way of looking at nutrient doses. It is the "highest average daily nutrient intake level that is likely to pose no risk of adverse health effects to almost all individuals in the general population."[3] For example, the level for vitamin D is 4,000 IU. That does not mean that higher doses are unsafe; they simply have not yet been studied. I find this more useful than the RDA because the former focuses on advising safe doses, which allows for higher-level doses. Remember, unlike with drugs, insufficient nutrient intake can cause severe side effects.

In addition to taking enough of the supplements you need, make sure you choose a good-quality supplement brand. Supplements should be chosen based on purity, potency, and dependable absorbability. It turns out that just because you swallow enough of a required supplement doesn't mean your body absorbs and uses all of it. A study in 2006 at the University of Alberta looked at how well different supplement brands dissolve when digested, which is important for nutrient absorption. The results were disappointing, and a number of products from reputable companies did not dissolve quickly enough to be absorbed in the bowel.[4] Most of the expensive supplements that I was taking at the time failed the test. Some supplement companies voluntarily follow standards of manufacturing called Good Manufacturing Practices (GMP) and International Organization for Standardization (ISO) standards,[5] which provide a level of quality assurance, but this is not required in all jurisdictions. There are also independent laboratories that certify products and compare contents to their companies' claims. These laboratories require companies to submit their products for analysis. It is a further step in quality assurance, and only a few companies bother with this.[6]

Essential Nutrients and Multivitamins

The Merck Manual of Diagnosis and Therapy, a reference guide widely used by the medical community, lists forty-five essential nutrients, meaning nutrients we have to get from food or supplements because we can't make them ourselves. In our modern times, however, these essential nutrients are harder and harder to find in food. We have developed the habit of growing food on the same land again and again, over hundreds of years, and we replenish only some of the nutrients depleted each time a crop grows. Therefore, our modern foods have less nutrient density than our ancestors' foods did.[7] Our intake of most vitamins, minerals, and phytochemicals is typically one and a half to eight times lower now than it was in the past. We do get more sodium and sugar,[8] but those two nutrients are harmful to our health when taken in excess. We also process much of our food, which further lowers its nutritional value. As mentioned in chapter 4, some of our foods are so overprocessed that they cannot rightly be called food. We are looking after our caloric needs but not our nutrient needs.[9] In addition, many of the drugs we take and the chemicals we are exposed to in our environment deplete the nutrients in our bodies.[10] For this reason, a balanced multivitamin and mineral supplement is a good insurance policy — it ensures we get at least some essential nutrients every day. Balanced vitamins and minerals are important for everyone, but they are most important for those on the road to recovery.[12]

TELOMERE PRESERVATION

There is research looking into the specifics of how nutritional supplementation can protect the immune system and possibly even preserve telomere length.[11] (Telomeres are discussed in chapter 5.)

Multivitamins are a mixture of vitamin A, B, C, D, E, K, all the essential minerals, and usually some other antioxidants. A multivitamin is like a general contractor. When you are building a house, the general contractor makes sure the materials needed to build a strong house are at the work site in sufficient quantities. That way, 2 x 2s won't be used to support a load-bearing wall. We are each made of an estimated 50 to 100 trillion cells, and while we may look the same every day, we actually change a lot; we make billions of new cells each day.[13] That is a ton of construction! If the optimal raw materials for the types of cells being built are not available, the new cells are not built as robust and resilient as they could be. For example, vitamin B_{12} and iron deficiencies cause the body to make substandard red blood cells. These poor-quality cells don't do their job well and they die prematurely. Taking multivitamins ensures your body gets at least some of all needed raw materials every day.[14]

Multivitamins are becoming more and more accepted by conventional medicine, and even the *Journal of the American Medical Association*, a highly conventional publication, has printed articles endorsing the use of multivitamin products.[15]

Antioxidants

Antioxidants are needed to curb free radicals. As we discussed in chapter 4, free radicals, such as ROS, are high-energy particles that come from our environment as well as being produced by our bodies during normal metabolic processes. If uncontrolled, free radicals cause unhealthy inflammation and damage to our tissues. If this damage accumulates, it plays a role in degenerative diseases. Antioxidants control free radicals by contributing electrons to them or to the tissues that were damaged by them. It is estimated that each of our cells takes many millions of "hits" from free radicals every day. Antioxidants taken in foods and supplements heal the damage from these hits. Antioxidants also have beneficial effects on blood pressure, sugar and fat metabolism, and heart health.[16]

Vitamins

Vitamin A is a fat-soluble vitamin, also called retinol, needed for healthy eyes and the detoxification of toxics such as dioxin and polychlorinated biphenyl (PCBs), which are especially harmful carcinogens. There have been some recent concerns that retinol may interfere with the metabolism of vitamin D and negate some of the health benefits of vitamin D. A safer option for supplementing vitamin A is beta-carotene. Beta-carotene is a precursor of vitamin A, and the body naturally turns it into vitamin A. It is water soluble and does not accumulate in our tissues and so, for most people, does not have negative effects.[17] Zinc is needed for vitamin A to function properly.[18]

Carotenoids are a large class of antioxidants derived from plants. Some carotenoids can be used by the body to produce vitamin A. Carotenoids have not been shown to interfere with vitamin D. They are mostly colorful compounds — red, orange, and yellow. They scavenge free radicals very well and help prevent the fats in our body from oxidizing and turning from helpful molecules into harmful ones. The carotenoids include alpha-carotene, beta-carotene, lycopene, lutein, astaxanthin, cryptoxanthin, and zeaxanthin, among others. As mentioned in chapter 4, when beta-carotene was studied on its own, like a drug, the results were disappointing. Carotenoids are likely best in combination with one another. They are a useful part of a multivitamin.

B vitamins are eight related, water-soluble vitamins. They are often found together in the same foods and are best taken this way, as B-complex vitamins. They are cofactors for enzymes, meaning they help our enzymes work properly. B vitamins support the health of our immune system, nervous system, red blood cells, skin, and muscles. They are needed for energy production and detoxification. B-complex vitamins with magnesium can be helpful for treating leg cramps and restless leg syndrome,[19] and taking extra B vitamins helps us deal with stress of all kinds.

Sometimes it is important to take one or more of the B vitamins separately — in particular, B_6, B_{12}, and folic acid. This trio reduces homocysteine, which can cause problems in our capillaries and increase our risk of heart disease. High homocysteine may also cause muscle pain.[20] B_6 can be used to reduce swelling in the body, and specifically to treat carpal tunnel syndrome. It also acts as a mild diuretic. Additionally, B_6 can be used by women during premenstruation to reduce puffiness, help with breast pain, and reduce overall symptoms of PMS.[21] Vitamin B_2 is helpful for migraines.[22]

B_{12} helps create red blood cells and maintain bone density. It also plays an important role in the health of our brain and nerves. In addition, a recent study shows it plays a specific role in pain. The study found that patients who receive daily B_{12} injections have reduced pain, even if their blood tests show they have normal levels of the vitamin.[23] The gut is not a reliable place to absorb B_{12}, so I recommend sublingual pills, meaning pills that sit and dissolve under the tongue. From there, they absorb straight into the bloodstream. In my experience, B_{12} injections work better in the short run, but it's best to switch to sublingual for the long term. Antacids interfere with the absorption of B_{12} from food. Be aware, B_{12} deficiency may not fully show on blood tests, and extreme deficiency is associated with pain and puzzling, even bizarre, neurologic symptoms.

Vitamin C is a powerful antioxidant. It is needed to build and repair collagen, which makes up our connective tissues, such as tendons, ligaments, and fascia.[24] It is also needed to build and repair muscles and bones. I recommend the form of vitamin C called L-ascorbate. Ascorbate helps make some of our stress hormones and neurotransmitters, and it supports our immune system.[25] It plays a role in mitochondrial energy production and helps to rid our body of toxic heavy metals.[26] Most other animals can make their own vitamin C from glucose. Humans cannot. Our vitamin C needs vary from day to day depending on stress, injury, and sickness.

Vitamin D is important for the function of over two hundred genes in the body.[27] It boosts the immune system, helps it fight infections like the flu, and reduces autoimmunity, a condition in which your immune system attacks its own body.[28] Vitamin D also plays a role in blood sugar metabolism and preventing diabetes.[29] Vitamin D helps our bones absorb calcium and improves muscle strength.[30] Childhood deficiency of vitamin D causes rickets, while in adults, long-term deficiency causes osteopenia and osteoporosis and raises certain cancer risks. Vitamin D deficiency is associated with pain.[31]

Most people in most areas of the Northern Hemisphere are vitamin D deficient.[32] When I practiced in Toronto, 95 percent of the patients I tested for vitamin D were profoundly deficient. I figured it would be less of a problem for my pain patients in Arizona, who are constantly in the sun. On checking their blood tests, however, I found 85 percent were profoundly deficient. The problem is that we are used to wearing sunscreen and hiding from the sun. Even when we do get exposed and form fat-soluble vitamin D on our skin, we wash it away before it can be fully absorbed.[33] When birds and animals are exposed to the sun and form vitamin D on their fur or feathers, they preen or groom themselves to ingest it. Humans tend to groom differently, which loses us much of this precious vitamin. Additionally, an unhealthy gut may have problems absorbing vitamin D in general, even D supplements.

Vitamin D is the "sunshine vitamin" and is not found in fruits or vegetables. There is some in fish. Vitamin D_3 is the form most usable by the body, but D_2 is good too. The marker for vitamin D status is 25-hydroxyvitamin-D [25(OH)D]. The only way to know your level of vitamin D is to have a blood test for 25OH vitamin D. You need an initial test and, if you are deficient, you need to be retested after a few months of taking a high dose of the supplement. Some people need only a small dose of 1,000 IU per day, while others need much more. Many authorities agree that optimal levels are in the higher part of the normal range. After your test, ask your doctor what your level is, since people are often told the level is normal when it is barely in the normal range. Some labs define normal as starting at 20 ng/ml (nanograms per milliliter is the US unit of measurement, while most of the rest of the world uses nanomoles per liter — nmol/l), but most experts think 30 ng/ml is the lowest acceptable level and many prefer levels above 40 ng/ml. The following table shows classifications of different levels of vitamin D in the United States and other countries.[34]

Table of Values for Assessing Vitamin D Status		
LEVEL OF 25(OH)D	UNITED STATES	MOST OTHER COUNTRIES
Deficient	0–40 ng/ml	0–100 nmol/l
Sufficient	40–80 ng/ml	100–200 nmol/l
Toxic	> 150 ng/ml	> 375 nmol/l

When I was in medical school, I was explicitly taught that vitamin D was potentially dangerous and that only very tiny doses were safe. Research over the past fifteen to twenty years has shown how wrong that information was. I have met with many authorities on nutritional research and asked them about the evidence supporting the alarmist statements I heard in medical school. As it turns out, there was never any evidence.

Natural vitamin E is made up of eight separate nutrients called tocopherols and tocotrienols. Synthetic vitamin E is usually labeled dl-alpha-tocopherol, and it does not have the same beneficial effect as the natural vitamin. A few studies have shown that vitamin E supplements have no benefit or even that they cause harm. These studies, however, were done using the synthetic vitamin containing only alpha-tocopherol; they included no gamma-tocopherol, the type that is particularly beneficial for the heart. Vitamin E is a powerful antioxidant and is being studied for its effect on the heart, the nervous system, and cancer development. It plays

A WINNING PRESCRIPTION

In 2009, the Chicago Blackhawks' physicians diagnosed most of the players with vitamin D deficiency and began a supplementation program with an average of 5,000 IU per day per player[35] The Hawks took the Western Division Championship that year. Earlier in the season, they had not been expected to do so.

a role in cell signaling, gene expression, and maintaining healthy cell membranes,[36] which are important for keeping cells healthy and durable when stressed.

Vitamin K is needed for bone development and the formation of the components of our blood responsible for clotting. Vitamin K is fat soluble. It should be in your multivitamin.

Minerals

Minerals come from the earth. Our bodies must ingest them and cannot make them. Fruits, vegetables, seeds, and nuts are good sources of minerals.

Calcium is probably the most commonly recommended mineral. Advertisers' focus on calcium for bones over the past decades has had its effect: everybody is fixated on calcium, thinking that more is better. In fact, balance is most important, and too much calcium can be harmful. Excess calcium has been associated with increased rates of heart disease.[37] Our bones are the storage reservoir for calcium, and they help the body maintain a balance of calcium in the blood. But other nutrients, too, affect bone density, including healthy oils, sufficient but not excessive protein, vitamins D and K, magnesium, phosphorus, and likely many other minerals. Exercise and hormone balance are also needed for healthy bones.

Calcium is needed for muscles to contract, blood to clot, and some neurotransmitters to function. Adequate calcium levels may also help prevent accumulation of lead in tissues. Normally adults need 1,000 mg from all sources — food and supplements. More is needed during pregnancy. Smoking; excess alcohol, caffeine, and salt consumption; a diet too high in protein or fiber; and hormonal imbalances all interfere with calcium levels.

Magnesium is needed by the body to make energy and is involved in over three hundred essential metabolic reactions.[38] It keeps bones strong, helps regulate blood sugar,[39] and controls the rate of nerve firing. It causes muscles to relax and so is helpful for cramps, spasms, and tight, painful muscles in general. It also reduces blood pressure, palpitations, and the frequency of migraines.[40] Magnesium can help irritable bowel syndrome by relaxing the gut muscles, reducing cramps, and relieving constipation.[41] It can improve sleep and reduce pain.[42]

Only 1 percent of the magnesium in your body is found in blood. The rest is found in tissues, making it difficult to measure. Although blood tests may not show magnesium deficiencies, it is one of the most common deficiencies in Western society.[43]

The primitive diet of our ancestors contained much more magnesium than ours does today. You can increase magnesium in your diet by eating nuts, seeds, lima beans, rice, molasses, dark chocolate, and dark leafy green vegetables and by drinking vegetable juice. The citrate, ascorbate, and glycinate forms of magnesium are best absorbed and utilized by the body.[44] If you have kidney disease, do not take extra magnesium before consulting your doctor. There is, however, research that suggests magnesium oxide prevents kidney stones.[45]

Generally, your body absorbs the magnesium it needs and leaves the excess in the bowel. If you take too much, you may experience diarrhea. I usually recommend that people take magnesium to bowel tolerance — that is, as much as your bowel tolerates without causing diarrhea. Some people do not tolerate magnesium well and get diarrhea from even very small amounts of additional magnesium. Let your symptoms guide you.

Sodium, potassium, and chloride are essential for life. They control the flow of water in and out of our cells. Sodium and potassium need to be balanced with each other, and they usually come combined with chloride. Table salt is sodium chloride, and many natural sea salts are a combination of sodium chloride and other mineral salts. There is way too much sodium in processed and restaurant foods — especially fast food. I have already discussed plenty of other reasons to avoid processed foods, and this is one more. The best sources of potassium are fruits and vegetables. Potassium supplements are fine in a multivitamin but should not be taken alone, unless you are on a drug that depletes you of potassium.

Chromium citrate has beneficial effects on blood sugar, insulin resistance, and type 2 diabetes.[46] Some industrial forms of chromium have been shown to cause cancer.

Iodine is essential for a healthy thyroid, which is the master gland that controls our metabolic rate and energy production. Many of our organs also need iodine. When I was a child, we used to get our scrapes painted with tincture of iodine. Since I almost never had uninjured knees until I was about twelve, I, like most of my peers, had adequate iodine and good thyroid function. There are now many other manufactured skin disinfectants on the market, and iodine is rarely used on scrapes and cuts. My children and subsequent generations have not had the benefit of getting their iodine levels topped off every time they fell.

Iodine levels in our food used to be higher as well. People used to clean the milk cows' udders with iodine and add iodine to cattle feed as a disinfectant. Now they use bromine to clean and antibiotics to disinfect. Bromine is toxic and antibiotics are causing a host of problems, which I cover in chapter 9.

I was taught in medical school that iodine is dangerous in all but tiny doses. The average Japanese woman, however, takes in 12.5 mg per day, and intakes can be as high as 60 mg in Japanese men — all from dietary sources. It's probably no coincidence that the Japanese have a very low rate of thyroid disease. In North America, we are told our daily intake should be from 150 to 290 micrograms.[47] (Since 1,000 micrograms make up 1 milligram, that is less than 1 mg.) There is a very big difference between the amount of iodine that the Japanese consume daily and the amount we are told is enough for us in North America.

There is a safe and simple test, one that requires more study, called the iodine skin test. (Do not do this test if you have an allergy to iodine.) To do this test, you use tincture of iodine to paint a patch about two inches square on your inner forearm or inner thigh. You can find tincture of iodine in the drugstore's first-aid section. Let the tincture dry, and it will leave an intense brownish yellow stain. If your body has enough iodine, the stain will be clearly visible twenty-four hours later. If you don't have enough iodine, your body will absorb what it needs and the stain will fade much faster. On pigmented skin, the stain will have a yellowish tinge. This test gives you a rough idea of your iodine level. There is a more precise but cumbersome test that calls for the patient to follow a specific diet for a week, get a "loading dose" of iodine, collect urine over a twenty-four-hour period, and have it analyzed. If all the patient's iodine intake is excreted, then his or her body has a lot of it; if only a small part of the ingested iodine comes out in the urine, then the body suffers from a deficiency.[48] The test depends on your diet at the time of the test. For the skin-test day wear dark clothes, since iodine stains will not come out.

It is best to get our iodine from natural food sources such as fish, kelp granules, and seaweed. The seas and oceans contain a lot of iodine, so swimming in the sea also works to replenish iodine. Many of my patients have asked if I could give them a prescription to go to the Caribbean. I wish I could.

Iron is essential for the formation of hemoglobin, the oxygen-carrying component of our red blood cells. Our cells need iron to produce energy, and iron deficiency is associated with fatigue. Iron also helps neutralize free radicals and is needed for growth, reproduction, healing, and immune health. Adequate iron reduces the absorption of lead from the intestine, so iron deficiency increases the risk of lead toxicity. In addition, the liver enzymes that detoxify and metabolize drugs and pollutants use iron.

Men need to absorb 1 mg of iron per day, and women in their childbearing years need about 2 mg. Athletes, teenagers, and pregnant and nursing moms have higher needs. Only a small amount of ingested iron is absorbed, and most women cannot consume enough food to absorb 2 mg. Therefore, supplements are often necessary. Iron is best absorbed if taken with some vitamin C.

In spite of the importance of iron for the body, iron can also be dangerous, and I do not recommend a multivitamin that contains iron.[49] Too much iron from supplementation can cause iron overload and is unhealthy for our organs, especially the heart. Iron from supplements and diet is especially dangerous in those who have a genetic disorder called hemochromatosis, a not uncommon, but potentially very serious, condition.

Trace minerals are required in tiny amounts. We know only a few of their functions in the body, and new roles are still being discovered. We can get many of them from fresh foods, and some supplements contain them as well.

Supplements to Reduce Pain

Glucosamine is widely recommended for joint health. Studies on glucosamine are inconsistent, but some well-done studies suggest it slows down the degeneration of cartilage in joints and reduces joint pain. It is commonly used to treat dogs and is an accepted joint therapy for horses.

Methylsulfonylmethane (MSM) is an anti-inflammatory molecule that contains sulfur. Sulfur is essential for making good-quality collagen, which is the foundation of our connective tissue, fascia, and bones. Research on MSM is not yet conclusive, but like glucosamine, it is accepted as helpful for horses.

Chondroitin is a long string of glucosamine molecules, and it too has some mixed reviews. I can't see why this form of glucosamine would be more helpful. It is a large molecule and is likely more difficult for us to digest and absorb.

Omega-3 fish oils — docosahexaenoic acid (DHA) and eicosapentaenoic acid (EPA) — are mostly found in fish oil, krill oil, fish, and seafood. Research shows omega-3s help a wide variety of painful conditions, including osteoarthritis, rheumatoid arthritis, dysmenorrhea, and inflammatory bowel disease.[50] They also may reduce the risk of other inflammatory, degenerative diseases, such as cardiovascular disease, diabetes, and some degenerative brain diseases. Omega-3s have been shown to reduce depression as well. It is important to get these oils from products that are not contaminated with heavy metals and other toxics.

Microdistilled fish oils are filtered for toxics, and their contents are usually at least 50 percent DHA and EPA.[51] High doses are sometimes needed, but consult your health care professional before taking large quantities. Another omega-3 oil, alpha-linolenic acid, can be found in flax and chia seeds and is very healthy. There are many beneficial nutrients in flax and chia seeds, and I suggest taking chia seeds or ground flax daily.

Most omega-6 oils promote inflammation. Our Western diet generally is high is omega-6s and low in omega-3s. This imbalance encourages inflammation in our bodies. The Linus Pauling Institute at the University of Oregon estimates that the ratio of omega-6 to omega-3 oils in the diet of early humans was one to one. The typical Western diet contains tons of vegetable oil and little fish, which is probably why our ratio of omega-6s to omega-3s is almost ten to one.[52]

Turmeric is a powerful anti-inflammatory that can be used for many types of pain.

S-adenosylmethionine (SAMe) is a molecule found naturally in the body and can also be taken as a dietary supplement. There are some studies showing SAMe performs as well as the prescription anti-inflammatories and gives similar joint pain relief and improved joint function. Of course, SAMe has fewer side effects and is generally considered safe. There is too little research, however, for me to strongly recommend it.[53]

Butterbur is a shrub. Studies show it is effective at preventing migraines and treating allergy symptoms.[54] The raw, unprocessed butterbur plant contains chemicals called pyrrolizidine alkaloids. Because these can cause liver damage, only butterbur products that have been properly processed and are labeled or certified as being free of pyrrolizidine alkaloids should be used. The Canadian Headache Society recommends standardized extract of butterbur for migraine prevention.

WHERE TO BEGIN WITH SUPPLEMENTS FOR PAIN

It may seem overwhelming to look at a long list of potential supplements and wonder how to start. My usual recommendation is to start with ensuring you have adequate vitamin D by doing a test and then supplementing as needed. I ask people to add magnesium, as well as omega-3 from fish or krill oil.

Support for Your Digestion

Probiotics, as discussed in chapter 4, are beneficial bacteria that help to maintain our gut health. Acidophilus and bifidus are the two main classes of probiotics, and if you use probiotic supplements, you should make sure both are present. Fructooligosaccharides (FOS) and inulin are two sources of prebiotics, which help probiotics thrive. A recent study found that African children have a greater variety of healthy bacteria in their guts, while European children on a Western diet have more of a particular bacteria called firmicutes, which is associated with obesity, autoimmune diseases, and allergies.[55]

Fiber is very important for the health of your gut. It gives bulk to bowel movements and traps toxics. The average American gets less than half the recommended 25 to 38 grams of fiber every day.[56] Fruits, vegetables, nuts, and seeds are excellent sources of fiber. Flaxseeds and psyllium husks are also good. Try to avoid getting your fiber from processed products that have sugar or artificial sweeteners.

Digestive enzymes can help your digestion by breaking down your food and making it easier for you to absorb nutrients. Proteolytic enzymes are a type of digestive enzymes that have been shown to relieve pain and speed up healing. A German study compared these enzymes to a prescription anti-inflammatory medication when treating patients with painful osteoarthritis of the hip.[57] They found that patients treated with enzymes had results comparable to those of patients treated with the prescription drug, except that those on enzymes didn't have the increased risk of heart attack and ulcers.[58] Bromelain, a digestive enzyme derived from pineapples, is being studied for its analgesic and anti-inflammatory effects.[59]

Hydrochloric acid is the type of acid we have in our stomach. It is very powerful and plays an important role in digestion and maintaining our overall health. Heartburn is usually caused by too much acid in the wrong place, but it may also be caused by not enough.[60] If the latter situation is yours, supplementing with hydrochloric acid can help. You should work with a knowledgeable health care professional to find out your specific needs.

The allium family, which includes garlic and onion, plays a significant role in gastrointestinal health and helps regulate blood sugar. The active ingredients in garlic are liberated when you crush or chop it and expose it to the air for a few minutes. Garlic and onions provide us with sulfur, which is needed for making and healing collagen, the main structural protein of our connective tissue. They are anti-infectives that kill harmful organisms while leaving friendly ones in our system, creating a healthy balance.

Deglycyrrhizinated licorice and *aloe vera* are both stomach remedies that can be used to treat an upset stomach and heartburn. If you have been diagnosed with ulcers, bleeding ulcers, or digestive cancers, consult your health care professional before you self-treat.

Peppermint oil is a safe and effective treatment for irritable bowel syndrome and chronic abdominal pain. Studies show it is as effective as drugs at treating these conditions. Naturally, peppermint oil has fewer serious side effects.[61]

Ginger has many uses. Fortunately, it's very tasty. It helps the stomach speed up digestion.[62] Ginger is also anti-inflammatory and has been shown to improve pain caused by osteoarthritis.[63] Ginger is a source of sulfur as well.

Support for Your Oxidative Stress System

L-glutamine is one of the amino acids, which are building blocks used to make protein. It is the most abundant amino acid in the body. High concentrations of L-glutamine are found in the brain, muscles, heart, lungs, kidney, liver, and gut lining. It is a source of energy and heals mucous membranes, including the lining of the mouth and digestive tract.[64] L-glutamine may improve neuropathic pain caused by chemotherapy.[65] It helps the body produce antioxidants but is not itself an antioxidant.[66]

Quercetin is a plant-based flavonoid and can come from grapes and pine bark. It helps oxidative stress and pain and is anti-inflammatory.[67]

CoQ$_{10}$ is produced by our cells. It can also be ingested from animal products and, to a lesser extent, from vegetables, seeds, and nuts. It is required by mitochondria, the energy factories of our cells. Muscle cells have a very large number of mitochondria and require a lot of energy for proper functioning. Some drugs, such as statins, interfere with the production of CoQ$_{10}$. This can cause muscle pain. Supplementing CoQ$_{10}$ can help, and it is also a powerful antioxidant capable of deactivating free radicals.

Resveratrol is an antioxidant with specific benefits for the heart. It may play a role in pain, and while it is not yet clear how it works, there are several proposed mechanisms.[68] Resveratrol has been shown to prevent inflammation and modify the stress response. You can find resveratrol as an oral supplement or cream. Studies are being done on injectable resveratrol, which is not yet ready for use on humans.

Melatonin is a hormone our body produces during sleep. It is also a powerful antioxidant. When used as a sleep aid, it is not addictive and does not disturb the natural rhythm of sleep as most sleep drugs do. Very small doses can be effective, so start with a low dose and gradually increase to find the dose that works best for you. Melatonin causes some people to have vivid dreams.

Support for Your Liver

The liver is one of the major systems responsible for detoxifying harmful substances in our body. These substances may come from our external environment or may be generated internally by our metabolism. There are many reactions involved in the process of detoxification, and sometimes the liver produces intermediate chemicals along the way. These intermediate chemicals can be toxic.

Virtually everything we ingest enters the liver. Some of it passes through unchanged, some is repurposed, and some is detoxified. Two types of enzymes, called phase I and phase II enzymes, are responsible for these activities. Phase I enzymes repurpose substances to be neutral, helpful, or toxic, and phase II enzymes detoxify substances, preparing them for excretion. If both types of enzymes are balanced, the process works well and all toxics are neutralized and eliminated. Keeping our phase II enzymes balanced can be tricky, as they need to be frequently replenished with the antioxidants glutathione and superoxide dismutase and with methylation. If we don't replenish them, phase II enzymes get overwhelmed by incoming toxics. This bottlenecks the detoxification process and can lead to cell damage by toxics and free radicals.

Liver support nutrients help to replenish superoxide dismutase and glutathione. The following are commonly found in products to promote liver health:

Silymarin is an extract of milk thistle fruits and seeds and of artichokes. Milk thistle has been used as a medicinal herb for over two thousand years. Silymarin increases glutathione and is anti-inflammatory. Studies have shown that silymarin can block the absorption of certain toxics and improves liver function in the case of most liver diseases, except for viral hepatitis.[69]

N-acetylcysteine (NAC) protects the body against a wide variety of toxics, stimulates phase II enzymes, disarms free radicals, and repairs damaged DNA. It also helps the liver produce glutathione. In addition, N-acetylcysteine binds metals into complexes so they can be excreted from the body. It is used in emergency rooms to treat acute poisoning from acetaminophen.

Alpha-lipoic acid is an antioxidant responsible for recycling other antioxidants. It prevents lipid peroxidation, which is damage to lipids in the body. It also helps glucose enter muscle cells, where it is used as energy, improves blood sugar by protecting insulin-producing cells in the pancreas, and protects nerve cells. Additionally, athletes use it to alleviate stress caused by exercise, and it is being studied as a chelator of heavy metals.[70]

Indole-3-carbinol and *isothiocyanates* are sulfur-containing chemicals found in cruciferous vegetables such as cabbage, brussels sprouts, cauliflower, collards, and broccoli. Both indole-3-carbinol and isothio-cyanates are antioxidants and are believed to stimulate the production of natural, detoxifying enzymes in the body, including phase I and II liver enzymes. These compounds are partially responsible for the lowered risk of cancer associated with eating cruciferous vegetables. They also reduce estrogen dominance by enhancing the body's metabolism of estrogens.

CHAPTER 8

EXERCISE

A bear, however hard he tries, grows tubby without exercise.

— A. A. MILNE, *Winnie-the-Pooh*

Our muscles were designed for movement. In the Western world, we spend much of our days in the same static postures, doing repetitive movements, usually with our arms. These habits get set early. Our children spend their time at school sitting with their heads bent over books and computers. Physical education classes are no longer mandatory in many areas, and often extracurricular activities involve more static postures and repetitive motion. In days gone by, we did chores every day that required more of our muscle groups. We had to grow our food, or at least shop for it regularly because refrigeration was a luxury few could afford. We chopped wood, hauled water, washed clothes by hand, and walked almost everywhere. Now we have automated heating systems and indoor plumbing, and we drive from activity to activity. Some of us are conscientious about getting daily exercise, but some of us are not.

I recommend at least thirty to forty-five minutes of aerobic exercise, four or five times per week. This helps weight control, cardiovascular health, energy levels, and mood. Exercise raises the level of your natural painkillers called endorphins, reduces body inflammation and insulin resistance, and normalizes blood sugar. The dynamic pumping action of working muscles improves circulation, which promotes oxygen delivery and the removal of toxins from our tissues. Regular exercise is one of the best prescriptions for people with chronic pain, fibromyalgia, depression, anxiety, insulin resistance, or diabetes.

Walking is an excellent exercise and requires no equipment. Swimming, biking, running, and the use of exercise machines such as treadmills, rowing machines, and elliptical trainers are also useful forms of aerobic exercise. Even if part of your body is in pain, it is worthwhile exercising the rest of your body. For example, if you have sore arms and are limited in your ability to exercise them, it is still valuable to do a lower-body workout. Exercise in general is beneficial for your entire body.

Muscle Memory

While the subject has not been adequately researched by the clinical scientific community, athletes and therapists understand that muscles have memories. Muscle memory means that muscles remember their good and bad experiences.[1] The consequences of this are tremendous for athletes, who, by constantly repeating an action, can train groups of muscles to automatically perform in a specific pattern. Some examples of this are a tennis player serving or a swimmer doing the breaststroke. Musicians achieve a similar effect when they practice their instruments.

Besides remembering a specific movement pattern, your muscles also remember their condition. For example, while an athlete's muscles change in size and composition when he stops exercising, his muscles will never forget their former condition. Even after a long period of inactivity, that athlete's muscles will get back in shape with much less training than it would take for muscles that were never in shape. The same can be said of injuries: muscles will revert to an injured state with less punishment or strain than was required the first time.[2] In general, this is good news. When you exercise regularly, your muscles change in a long-lasting way.

Some Therapeutic Exercises

Movement therapies are gentle exercises meant to curb unhelpful daily movements by retraining our movement patterns. Many of us have had injuries without realizing how they change our movement patterns. For example, after an injury we may not swing our arms equally, we may tilt slightly to one side, or we may have contracted muscles that twist or shift our spine. Sometimes, we develop these patterns through habits or through injuries that don't fully heal. Movement therapies identify and improve our awareness of unhealthy patterns and restore better ones. These therapies respect the interconnectedness of our body parts — upper and lower, right and left. The exercises involved are sometimes only very small movements. They are so gentle that even very injured people can work with them. There are several different schools of movement therapies to choose from, including Feldenkrais, Alexander, Mitzvah, Trager, and Laban-Bartenieff. All of these techniques can reduce pain and restore health.

HURT DOES NOT MEAN HARM

Sometimes people in pain are fearful of moving their bodies. But without movement, you won't get better. It is important to understand the difference between hurt and harm. Hurt is pain that is not causing damage to your tissues. Harm is pain that signals damage. If you have a sore back and move around, you may experience additional pain. But in most cases that pain is not causing damage. In the long run it will not make you worse, but it will help you heal. You need to work with a professional, such as a physical therapist, who will guide you.

Pilates is a system of exercise developed by Joseph Hubertus Pilates in the early twentieth century. It has since become popular — first in dance communities in Europe and then in North America. Pilates keeps the body aligned using core strength — the strength of the postural muscles in the abdomen and the upper back. It develops body awareness and proper posture while promoting flexibility and strength. Pilates is useful for injured and novice exercisers as well as for those with very high fitness levels.

Combination workouts using Pilates and exercise balls are becoming popular as well. Exercise balls can be used as an aid for stretching and strengthening and to add fun to a workout. They are inexpensive and have tremendous versatility. They strengthen core muscles and are useful for balance.[3] Some people sit on them at work for a change from seated-chair postures.

Yoga dates back more than five thousand years. Studies show it can improve flexibility, strength, and stamina. Using yoga, some people can achieve fitness levels that are equal to or higher than those of people who use only conventional exercises like running and weight lifting. It also decreases pain and improves function in pain patients. As with any therapy, however, if you are injured, then care, patience, and experience are needed. If you have injuries, it is important to work with an instructor who understands injuries and knows how to modify your exercises appropriately. Regardless, don't let experienced yogis discourage you. The intention of a yoga pose is more important than the actual position achieved. Not everyone needs to look like a pretzel. The National Institutes of Health website has a good summary of yoga research.[4]

Tai chi and qi gong also offer a combination of stretch and strength exercises and can be used by pain patients. Yoga, tai chi, and qi gong are all moving meditations and benefit both the mind and the body.[5]

Aqua jogging is doing running movements in water. It can be useful for individuals of all fitness levels, even high-level athletes. In water, buoyancy makes our bodies feel lighter and allows us freer movement. This is especially helpful for those with joint pain. When you move in water, you always experience gentle resistance. As a result, water is a great place to begin gentle strengthening. Very weak or debilitated individuals can exercise in water using a flotation belt.

Stretchy bands are an inexpensive way to develop muscle strength. They are portable and therefore convenient for traveling.

Tabata, developed by a gymnast of the same name, is interval training exercise using light weights. After her career in gymnastics, Tabata became an exercise physiologist and showed that this type of exercise, done for only four minutes every other day, speeds up the metabolism and burns calories for hours after the exercise is finished.

A rebounder is a minitrampoline. It can help you become fit. At first, depending on your condition, you may only be able to step onto it and gently bounce with your feet firmly planted on the mesh in the middle. This is still useful, because even this minimal movement improves circulation in your legs. As you get stronger, you can move your feet side to side or back and forth. Although the aim is not to jump high or to bring your feet far off the mesh, rebounding can still be a vigorous exercise. You may need to consult an exercise therapist or trainer to establish your program. Be careful not to fall off. I recommend using one with a hand bar for balance.

RECONDITIONING PAIN, OR NEW-INJURY PAIN?

Once you start your exercise program, your muscles may feel achy for a day or two. This is normal, and it is called reconditioning pain: your muscles have to get used to new activities. Sometimes you might worry that you are reinjuring yourself. How can you tell the difference? You should start with a level of exercise that feels easy. Then gradually increase the level of difficulty by increasing the resistance or the time spent. You might experience some pain after your workout. This can last a few days, but you should have less and less pain after each workout, until the next time you increase the intensity of your exercise. Then the aching feeling will return for a few days. This is called reconditioning pain and is normal and healthy.

If you feel more and more pain each time you exercise, you may be injuring yourself. If this is the case, you should consult your treatment team. They may need to adjust your exercises.

CHAPTER 9

PRESCRIPTION DRUGS

*Much of the scientific evidence that doctors rely upon to prescribe drugs
is more like infomercials than scientific evidence.*

— JOHN ABRAMSON, *Overdosed America*

Drugs that have been properly prescribed and properly taken are the
fourth-leading cause of death in North America. This is alarming
when you consider that most drugs don't actually fix anything — they
only relieve symptoms.[1] Taking drugs can be a little like releasing a bull
in a china shop. Doctors know the drug will do something to your system, but its effects on an individual can be quite unpredictable. This
is especially the case with chronic pain medications. The processes by
which pain develops in our system, and by which our system heals itself,
are very complicated. If any one part of these processes changes, all processes and our whole system are affected. This can mean more pain and
side effects. Oftentimes, chronic pain patients end up on a long list of

drugs that all cause bad side effects on their own, cause worse side effects when combined, and leave the patient worse off in the long run. Regarding drugs, the best advice I can give is: "Proceed with caution." Nature and time can be powerful healers, and I recommend, whenever possible, letting them work as they were intended to.

Fads

We would like to think a doctor chooses treatments based entirely on a patient's needs. Unfortunately, that is not always the case. Sometimes, medical treatments are dictated by fads, which could be based on a recent article, popularized research, a drug's availability, insurance billing, or even simply a charismatic doctor's decision. These fads are helpful when founded on sound science, but sometimes they are not.

In 1964, Robert A. Wilson wrote an article about hormone replacement therapy titled "No More Menopause." As a result of the article, published in *Newsweek*, estrogen replacement became very popular. Some doctors went so far as to recommend estrogen replacement to all menopausal women, whether or not they had troublesome menopausal symptoms. We have known since the 1930s that estrogen is carcinogenic, but researchers in the decades after Wilson's article had to prove it all over again before the fad would die. In the 1990s, a very large study called the Women's Health Initiative looked at the effects of these estrogen treatments. The women in the study suffered such a considerable increase in breast cancer that the study was halted early. The 1960s also saw a fad of using X-rays to treat acne. It was soon shown that X-rays cause thyroid cancers, and the trend stopped. Remarkably, there was never research that showed it was safe to treat acne with X-rays in the first place.

In the late 1990s, an anti-inflammatory drug called Vioxx was put on the market to treat pain and arthritis. It became hugely popular and generated sales of $2.5 billion a year. In 2000, a study was published showing that Vioxx increases the rate of heart attacks and stroke.[2] This did little to reduce its popularity. Then at a hearing in 2004, it was revealed that the company that produced Vioxx had known, even before it was approved for use, that low doses increase the risk of heart attack by nearly seven-fold. Despite this, the labeling at the time of FDA approval contained nothing about heart attack risks.[3] As a result of the 2004 hearings, Vioxx was withdrawn from the market, but even then the Vioxx fad was strong among physicians and patient groups who cried for it to be brought back. By that time, Vioxx had already caused an estimated 160,000 unnecessary heart attacks and strokes.[4]

Today, much of the medical community treats cholesterol as the sole cause of heart attacks. This has led to a fad of cholesterol-lowering drugs called statins, which I discussed in chapter 2. In truth, not everyone with high cholesterol gets a heart attack, and not everyone with low cholesterol is protected. Since the late 1970s, evidence has been mounting that the main causes of heart disease are our starchy, high-glycemic, overprocessed diets, which are high in calories and low in nutrition; our lack of physical activity; and our crazy, stressful lifestyles. It seems these factors cause insulin resistance and inflammation that in turn cause heart disease. The solution is lifestyle change, not a drug that changes cholesterol numbers but does nothing for other risks. Nevertheless, even doctors who acknowledge diet and lifestyle as important are caught up in the fad of prescribing drugs for cholesterol. Statins have become the "standard of care," meaning most of the medical community is pushing them. As a result, statins have been the top revenue drugs for most of the twenty-first century.[5]

Interestingly, the statin fad was not pulled from thin air. It is actually based on prevailing research. Prevailing research, however, does not necessarily mean good research or even honestly presented research. Sometimes research is conducted by organizations and individuals who have a vested interest in the outcome, like drug companies or the researchers getting paid directly by them. This was the case with statins, and the drug companies that researched statins presented only limited findings as important. For example, statin companies have often reported that the drug prevents a third of all heart attacks. This information is misleading, however, because it doesn't cover the "number needed to treat" — that is, the number of people who need to be treated to prevent one illness or unwanted event. For statins, the number is over one hundred. Therefore, more than one hundred people need to be treated with statins, over a period of many years, just to prevent one heart attack. That means at least ninety-nine people have to risk the side effects of statins to help one person. In this way, drug companies can create a fad by using prevailing research but focusing only on favorable numbers. Patients might think differently about many commonly used drugs and even surgeries if they knew their "numbers needed to treat."

Allopathic medicine likes organization. It requires categories for symptoms and names for diseases and conditions. As I mentioned in chapter 3, these names, or diagnoses, are useful because they streamline our thinking and expectations. Medical names, however, can also pro- mote unhelpful fads. For example, pain in the elbow from overuse was, for a long time, called tendinitis. The suffix *itis* in a medical word means "inflammation," which triggers doctors to prescribe anti-inflammatories. It turns out that anti-inflammatories don't actually help tendinitis very well — doctors were only prescribing them because of the name.[6] This condition is now called tendinosis. The suffix *osis* means "abnormal," which signals doctors to refer those patients for therapy.

The tendinitis example explains how a name, or diagnosis, can cause a fad of improper drug prescriptions. The opposite is also possible: a drug can cause a fad of improper diagnoses. Fibromyalgia (FM) is a con- fusing condition. It is not yet a disease with a clear cause. A diagnosis of FM is given to individuals who suffer from a collection of symptoms that probably arise from a wide variety of causes that still need to be explored. Recently, drugs were approved for use on FM patients. These drugs have been shown to help some people, some of the time. The side effects of these drugs can be nausea, constipation, weight gain, muscle pain, fatigue, dizziness, insomnia, and decreased sex drive. Alarmingly, since these drugs became available, FM diagnoses have become much more common. Doctors are so conditioned to prescribe drugs that they are more likely to diagnose a patient with FM because there are drugs approved to treat the disorder.

Drugs and Our Chemistry

When you take a drug, your body metabolizes it into related compounds called metabolites. Some of these metabolites are active, meaning they have an effect on us, and some are not. Sometimes the metabolites get processed several times into different substances before they are finally excreted from the body. Therefore, when you take a drug you may actually be introducing several new chemicals into your body, and not just the one you took in the pill. In addition, there may be extra chemicals in the pill, called fillers and excipients. All of these different substances can confuse your body — and they are all from just one drug. If you are prescribed more than one drug, all of their intended chemicals, their fillers, and the subsequent metabolites mix together to make even more compounds. Modern medicine has no way of telling what is really happening in that chemical soup. Doctors can look up how some major drugs interact, but a complete explanation is out of reach.

The liver is the main place in your body where drugs, toxins, poisons, and potential poisons get detoxified before eventually being excreted. The liver works hard to detoxify molecules that would otherwise build up to damaging levels. Some drugs can change the liver's process by changing certain enzymes it relies on. This can slow or speed up liver function, which can in turn slow or speed up the processing of drugs. As a result, it can be difficult to predict how long certain drugs will remain in your body. If you assume a drug is out of your system and it isn't, you can risk unintentionally mixing drugs. This makes it even harder to tell what is happening in that chemical soup.

Drugs work by changing the chemical reactions in your cells. For example, statins work by interfering with an enzyme, which then lowers cholesterol. Oftentimes, however, a drug changes a chemical reaction that has more than one role in the body. This is a cause of drug side effects. For example, the enzyme that statins interfere with is responsible not only for cholesterol but also for making an antioxidant called coenzyme Q_{10} (CoQ_{10}), which is needed to keep your muscle and nerve cells healthy. A deficiency of CoQ_{10} causes muscle pain and sometimes muscle breakdown. It can even cause heart attacks. In addition, statins have not been studied long enough for us to know the effect of lower CoQ_{10} levels on the brain. As another example, some anti-inflammatory drugs decrease inflammation in your injured knee but also interfere with how the stomach protects itself from stomach acid.

Placebos

All drugs work by changing chemical reactions in your cells, but not all the effects of drugs come from those changes. If you expect a drug to accomplish something, your body does too, and often whether or not the drug accomplishes those things chemically, your body works to fulfill those expectations on its own. This is called the placebo effect. For example, drinking decaffeinated coffee can sometimes keep you as alert as drinking regular coffee. There is much less caffeine in decaffeinated coffee, but your body doesn't actually need a drug or a chemical reaction to wake itself up — it's fully capable of doing that on its own. It just needs a prompt, and in this case that prompt is the taste or feeling of coffee.

The placebo effect happens so frequently that placebos are incorporated into all drug studies. In these studies, a placebo is a sham drug. It's a pill that has no active ingredient, causes no chemical reaction, and isn't a drug at all. It does nothing besides look and feel like a drug. In drug studies, placebos determine how much of a drug's effect is actually just the body fulfilling its own expectations — that is, how much is just the placebo effect. While everyone in these studies thinks they are receiving an actual drug, some are given only placebos, usually sugar pills. On average, of the people in these studies given only placebos, between 30 and 60 percent get better.

As it turns out, placebos can have an effect on patients even if they know they're taking them. In a recent study on irritable bowel syndrome, patients were treated only with placebos, and were told so.[7] Researchers explained to these patients that sometimes bowel pain improves with an inactive pill. Amazingly, many of them improved compared to a group that received no treatment.

Simply convincing people they can heal themselves seems to unleash the body's ability to do so. In this way, placebos are a measure of our body's ability to heal itself. They offer healing at no expense, with no risk of adverse effects or addiction. Sadly, allopathic medicine has a tendency to brush placebos aside as shams. Nevertheless, the placebo effect will always play a significant role in medicine. In fact, scientists estimate that 30 to 60 percent of the effect of all interventions — which includes drugs, surgery, and alternative practices — is the placebo effect.[8]

Drugs Used to Treat Pain

Many different categories of drugs are used in pain treatment.

Simple Analgesics, or Painkillers

Painkillers can relieve symptoms but do not help the body heal. While they can improve function, interrupt the cycle of pain, and simply give relief, they sometimes lead to rebound pain, which is an increase in pain after the drug is stopped. Rebound pain is common in headache and migraine patients, whose headaches return as soon as the dose wears off. These patients should not take painkillers — not even over-the-counter ones — regularly. In addition, some pain medications, if they are taken continuously, become less effective over time.

ACETAMINOPHEN

Acetaminophen can help with mild to moderate pain, and the manufacturers suggest an upper limit of 3,000 mg per day, which was just recently reduced from 4,000 mg. Many people assume that over-the-counter medications are harmless. This is not true, and acetaminophen can have some very dangerous side effects. Never take more than the recommended dose; and if you have liver or kidney disease, even the maximum recommended dose may be dangerous for you. In addition, some other over-the-counter medications contain acetaminophen. It's a good idea to check labels to avoid accidentally taking too much. The therapeutic dose, meaning the helpful dose, and the toxic dose of acetaminophen are not far apart. Be careful not to reach the toxic dose — it can cause severe liver damage. Consuming alcohol while taking acetaminophen can increase the risk of liver damage.

ASPIRIN

Aspirin, or acetylsalicylic acid, was created from salicin, a derivative of white willow bark, a plant long known to relieve fevers, inflammation, and pain. Salicin is slower to start working than aspirin is, but its effects last longer, and it doesn't cause the stomach side effects that aspirin does. Aspirin can cause ulcers and other damage to the lining of the digestive tract. With regular use, it can also cause long-term kidney damage. Aspirin set the stage for the development of nonsteroidal anti-inflammatories.

NONSTEROIDAL ANTI-INFLAMMATORIES

Nonsteroidal anti-inflammatories (NSAIDs) are also called anti-inflammatories. These drugs reduce inflammation by reducing the production of prostaglandins (PGs), which are hormone-like substances that have many functions in the body. There are different types of PGs, each of which has different and sometimes even opposite functions. PGs can contract or relax muscles in organs and blood vessels, increase or decrease cell growth, raise or lower blood pressure, cause inflammation or reduce it, and protect nerve cells or sensitize them. When you take an NSAID, it can interrupt the balance of PGs and so can change some or all of these functions. The disruption of PGs is one of the major causes of NSAID side effects, which mostly affect the gut and can cause stomach inflammation, bleeding digestive-system ulcers and leaky gut. Chronic use of these medications also affects kidney function and can cause chronic kidney failure. In addition, NSAIDs can cause you to retain fluids, which is dangerous for people with heart disease or high blood pressure. Patients who have already had a heart attack are now being cautioned to avoid all types of NSAIDs.[9] For these individuals, NSAIDs can greatly increase the risk of further heart attacks.[10]

People often assume that because they do not feel any stomach irritation while taking an NSAID, they are not at risk. Nevertheless, it is possible to suffer from stomach damage caused by NSAIDs without ever experiencing heartburn or stomach pain. A recent study examined this phenomenon by comparing twenty-one patients who used NSAIDs to twenty control patients who did not. After at least three months on NSAIDs, 71 percent of the patients had ulcers in the small bowel, compared to 10 percent of the controls. All of the patients were asymptomatic, meaning they had no symptoms or reason to suspect they had bowel damage. Antacids and stomach protectants can help reduce the occurrence of ulcers, but these too should be used with caution.

Current research is showing that NSAIDs, when used regularly, may interfere with the healing of fractures, delay healing in certain types of tendon injuries, and decrease bone density in men.[11] An older study also suggests that NSAIDs interfere with the repair of cartilage and so could worsen arthritis — the very condition they are often used to treat.[12]

Corticosteroids

Corticosteroids, sometimes simply called steroids,[13] can be used to treat painful conditions. These steroids can dramatically reduce inflammation, which can save lives in certain situations. For example, corticosteroids are very useful in treating life-threatening brain or throat swelling. They are also useful in treating some painful rheumatic conditions, such as giant cell arteritis, polymyalgia rheumatica, and rheumatoid arthritis. In these cases, corticosteroids can prevent blindness and joint or organ damage. They also reduce pain, but pain control is not the primary goal of the treatment.

While commonly done, using steroids to treat pain alone is usually a bad idea. Every cell in the body has receptors for corticosteroids, so their effects on the body are far-reaching. Possible side effects are severe and include bone loss, obesity, and changes in blood cholesterol and blood sugar. Sometimes corticosteroids can cause osteoporosis — which is the thinning of bones — and osteonecrosis, which is the death of bone structure, and which leads to bone collapse. Osteonecrosis most commonly occurs at the hip and has dangerous consequences. Corticosteroids can also cause hormone imbalances, depression, and anxiety. In addition, they can weaken the body's defense against certain infections.

Prednisone is the most commonly prescribed oral corticosteroid. When prednisone is taken, the body stores it in its fat tissues and then slowly releases it, which causes prolonged exposure to potential side effects.

There are several commonly prescribed injectable corticosteroids. They can be injected into painful areas around nerves and tendons or into muscles, joints, bursa, and other structures. Although this treatment can give pain relief and reduce inflammation, studies suggest the results are often disappointing. Injecting a painful area too frequently can cause tissue weakness, and steroid injections can lead to crystal formation.[14] Corticosteroids can also lead to muscle atrophy and can even make painful conditions worse. Injecting joints with steroids is a double-edged sword: the joint may become more comfortable but may degenerate faster in the long run. In the case of osteoarthritis caused by wear and tear, steroids may speed up the need for surgery. There are, however, exceptions — with inflammatory arthritis like rheumatoid arthritis, injectable corticosteroids are helpful and can delay surgery.

Hydrocortisone is another corticosteroid. It is the same molecule as a steroid our adrenal glands manufacture, and if corticosteroids are absolutely necessary, then taking this form in a twice-a-day dosage may be the safest option. Practitioners of integrative medicine sometimes prescribe hydrocortisone in physiological doses, meaning close to the amount the body would make on its own if it were perfectly healthy. This is only necessary if the adrenal glands are depleted or are producing hormones at the wrong time of day.[15] In these cases, hydrocortisone is used for a short time, until other health-promoting interventions, like diet, exercise, pain treatments, and sleep improvement, allow the body to normalize its own adrenal functions.

Opioids

Opioids are painkillers that come from the opium poppy plant. Synthetic opioids can also be made in a laboratory. Although heroin, a recreational opioid, was made illegal in 1924, opioids have long been accepted by the medical world as treatment for acute pain, such as pain caused by broken bones or surgery. For most of the twentieth century, however, opioids were avoided for treating most chronic pain — the exception was cancer pain. It was recognized that opioids were too dangerous to use over the long term. It was also recognized that patients who take opioids for extended periods develop a tolerance to them. For these patients, opioids become less effective and so patients need higher doses to achieve the same pain relief. In the case of cancer patients, increased doses were not as problematic — the patient's lives were likely to be shorter anyway. Doctors treating cancer patients would administer the required doses to keep their patients comfortable if the patients accepted the risks, including death, that the drug posed. Then suddenly in the 1990s, opioids began to be heavily promoted to treat chronic, noncancer pain. Advertisements and scientific papers alike began telling doctors that opioids were safe for chronic pain patients, and that when tolerance developed, it was safe to just keep increasing doses. At one point it was even said that people in pain don't get addicted.

The result was enthusiastic opioid prescribing in the United States. Today, America consumes fifty times more opioids than the rest of the world combined, and prescription opioids kill more Americans than illegal drugs do.[16] For patients on high doses of opioids, a glass of wine, a sleeping pill, or a cold could easily become deadly. Opioids affect the respiratory center of the brain and slow down our breathing. While they get less effective at relieving pain over time, they still present a risk due to our slowed breathing. Too often, patients taking high but properly prescribed doses simply stop breathing at night. In addition, chronic use and, most often, high doses of opioids can actually make pain worse. This is called hyperalgesia, and it results in pain from pressure or activities that should not normally be painful. Conditions that commonly result in hyperalgesia from regular opioid use include chronic low-back pain, FM, and chronic fatigue.

If used carefully and in low doses, opioids can sometimes be useful for chronic conditions. They should only be used in low doses, and for most patients they should not be used daily. In addition, once an effective dose is determined, the dose should never be increased — not even if it becomes less effective. The purpose of opioids in these cases is to improve function and to transition patients back to active, productive lives. By returning to normal daily habits, patients will find that their pain improves on its own — active daily habits release natural anti-inflammatories and endorphins, which, as I mentioned in chapter 8, are natural painkillers.

I have seen countless patients who have developed tolerance to opioids. At a certain point, they are all faced with a decision: up the dosage and accept the risks, or stop taking opioids and go through withdrawal. The side effects of withdrawal are so severe that many patients say they would not have started opioids if they had been better informed. Although the withdrawal period and the increased pain associated with it can last up to six months, most patients find that their level of pain drops afterward. At that time, surprisingly, patients often say that they have less pain than they experienced while on opioids, before withdrawal, or the same level of pain. Reducing or stopping opioids is always better than upping the dosage. In the end, reduced dosages often get patients more involved in regular activities and their families.

The possible side effects of opioids are too many to list here, but the most common ones are constipation, difficulty urinating, nausea, vomiting, itching, drowsiness, confusion, suppression of sex hormones leading to changes in menstrual periods and to impotence, abdominal and bowel pain, change in electrocardiogram results, poor memory and concentration, euphoria, flushing, and respiratory depression that can be life threatening.

FACTS ABOUT OPIOIDS

Tolerance: Over time, patients tend to develop tolerance to opioids, meaning the opioids lose their effectiveness and patients need higher doses to produce the same effects.

Dependence: When a patient's body adapts to opioids, it is called dependence. If that patient suddenly stops taking the drug, he will experience withdrawal symptoms.

Addiction: A patient with an opioid addiction craves the drug and has a continued impulse to take it, despite harmful consequences, which may be physical, mental, or social. About 15 percent of the population is genetically predisposed to addiction. One of the dangers of widely prescribing strong opioids is that we don't know who those susceptible individuals are. Prescribing opioids to someone genetically predisposed to addiction may change the course of her life dramatically.[17]

Hyperalgesia: Those who take opioids regularly, and especially those who take high doses, can experience a worsening of pain called hyperalgesia. This pain is caused by opioids and can last for up to six months after the drug is stopped. Patients with chronic, nonmalignant pain should discuss hyperalgesia with their doctors before taking opioids. These patients in particular are at risk of ending up in worse pain than they began with.

Opioid Antagonists

Most opioids are agonists, meaning they affect our cells by stimulating opioid receptor sites. A few opioids are antagonists, which affect our cells by blocking those same receptor sites. Sometimes tiny doses of opioid antagonists can affect pain that is unresponsive to opioid agonists. In addition, some opioids have both agonist and antagonist properties. Naltrexone is an opioid antagonist that is currently getting a lot of attention.

It is being used in tiny doses in a drug called low-dose naltrexone. It is thought that this drug quiets down part of the nervous system that gets overactivated and causes hyperalgesia.

Adjuvant Pain Therapies

Some pain drugs were not originally designed to treat pain, and so they are not part of the painkiller family. In these cases, pain relief was an unexpected side effect of the drug's initial purpose. For example, while antidepressants and anticonvulsants are sometimes used to treat pain, they were actually designed to treat depression and epilepsy. Some of these drugs are helpful on their own, and others work by boosting pain-killers — making painkillers work better or longer — and some work very well on particular types of pain.

Antidepressants

Depression has a symbiotic relationship with pain syndromes: depression aggravates pain, and chronic pain can cause depression. Depression should be treated through psychological therapy or a mind-body training course, and antidepressants should be used only when necessary, which is usually in cases of severe depression. Several new studies show that "mild to moderate" and "early severe" depressions do not benefit significantly from these drugs.[18]

Although many antidepressants have been found to affect pain, we don't fully understand how. We also don't yet understand their long-term effects on pain patients, or why they relieve pain better for some patients than for others. Fortunately, the doses needed for effective pain treatment can sometimes be very low, and in many cases antidepressants are needed only briefly or until the patient begins sleeping better, exercising regularly, and eating properly. In other cases, however, patients have to stay on the drug for the long term.

Tricyclics are an older class of antidepressants that affect many different neurotransmitters, including serotonin, noradrenaline, dopamine, and others. They have been labeled "dirty drugs" because they affect so many different systems. They are strong sedatives, and their possible side effects include dry mouth, blurred vision, difficulty urinating, and, rarely, movement disorders. Nevertheless, they can improve pain and sleep. I often prescribe tiny doses that need to be specially made by a pharmacist. Those with FM, chronic fatigue and immune dysfunction syndrome, or multiple chemical sensitivities are especially sensitive to tricyclics, and tiny doses are more than enough for them. Those individuals may get severe side effects from normal doses.

Selective serotonin reuptake inhibitors and serotonin-norepinephrine reuptake inhibitors are newer antidepressants. Their side effects, though fewer than those of tricyclics, include apathy, liver dysfunction, sexual dysfunction, and weight gain. They seem to be effective in about 25 percent of cases.[19]

Anticonvulsants

As mentioned earlier, anticonvulsants were designed to treat epilepsy, but they have also been found to improve pain. They are thought to work best on certain types of nerve pain, including pain in diabetics, smokers, and chemotherapy patients. These individuals are more prone to small-nerve damage, which often happens in their hands and feet but can also happen elsewhere. Anticonvulsants are widely used and for some conditions are highly effective.

Muscle Relaxants

Muscle relaxants can provide some patients with relief from muscle pain and spasms. There are, however, several different types of muscle relaxants, and some of the drugs used for this purpose are risky. As an example, benzodiazepines are sedatives, and some of them cause muscle relaxation. These drugs have a high risk of dependence and a long list of serious side effects. They are, consequently, no longer favored as muscle relaxants for chronic use. Another example is carisoprodol, which still sometimes gets used for muscle relaxation but carries a high risk of oversedation and addiction.

Cyclobenzaprine, baclofen, methocarbamol, and tizanidine are currently the most commonly used muscle relaxants. They are somewhat effective, but in most cases regular exercise and consistent stretching can probably do more for patients. This is not the case with baclofen, which is used for people who have extreme spasms or muscle contraction from multiple sclerosis, stroke, or cerebral palsy.

Sleep Medications

Drugs that affect sleep also affect pain; sleep deprivation worsens pain syndromes, and restful sleep encourages healing and the development of coping skills. There are many different types of sleep medications, many of which also belong to other drug categories. In fact, some of the most effective sleep medications with the best long-term safety records are antidepressants. Certain muscle relaxants are also considered sleep medications, including benzodiazepines. Benzodiazepines, however, also reduce the dream phase of sleep. When you stop taking the medication, you may find you dream more than usual, which can lead to feeling unrested. Of course, this adjustment period eventually wears off, and you shouldn't let it convince you that you actually need the drug.

Medications can also interfere with sleep. These medications can be found in many drug categories, including opioids, decongestants, heart medications, statins, antidepressants, asthma drugs, and stimulants to treat attention deficit disorder.

Antihistamines

Antihistamines are usually associated with the treatment of allergies or nausea. They control histamine, a proinflammatory molecule. Histamine molecules are produced throughout the body, and when released they cause swelling, redness, and pain. They also play a significant role in the balance of immune and inflammatory reactions. Today, antihistamines are not commonly used to treat pain, but there may be a role for them in the future. The older, sedating varieties help some people sleep. The newer, nonsedating ones may have an anti-inflammatory effect and could reduce bone pain caused by chemotherapy.[20]

Sympathetic Blockers

We discussed in chapter 5 how the sympathetic and parasympathetic nervous systems affect body functions and inflammation. They also play a significant role in pain. In the hands and feet, the sympathetic nervous system causes blood vessels to contract, causing those extremities to turn pale, mottled, and sometimes even red, purple, or blue. This can cause various levels of pain. If cases are severe they may be called Raynaud disease or syndrome. I have also seen this constriction of blood vessels associated with repetitive strain injuries, such as carpal tunnel syndrome, trigger finger, extensor and flexor tendinitis, and de Quervain's tenosynovitis. In these cases, drugs that block the sympathetic nervous system, called alpha blockers, can be used to relieve pain.[21] Alpha blockers help to restore circulation needed for healing. Patients usually need to use the medication regularly for a few months and then only periodically — when they are exposed to cold or experiencing a very stressful time. These drugs may also be useful in treating neuropathic pain.

Other Drugs That Can Reduce Pain

Calcium channel blockers are used to lower blood pressure. They do this by dilating the small blood vessels in your limbs. This leads to better circulation and the side effect of warmer hands and feet. For some people, this relieves pain in the hands and feet.

Doxycycline is a common antibiotic. It has been shown, in lab animals, to affect the glial and microglial cells, which play a role in the development of neuropathic pain. After I read the research on doxycycline, I had a few patients try it. The results were disappointing, and the area needs more research.

Bisphosphonates are drugs developed to improve bone density. They can be used to reduce bone pain from cancer.

Dextromethorphan is often found in cough syrups. In the laboratory, it was found to affect a particular type of pain receptors, called N-methyl-D-aspartate (NMDA) receptors. In practice, however, it has not been shown to have a significant effect on pain.

Quinine sulfate has been used to treat nighttime leg cramps. In the United States, however, it is no longer approved for this use. It can cause serious side effects, such as cardiac arrhythmias and blood disorders. *Vitamin B complex* and *magnesium* can also help these leg cramps, and they have fewer side effects. In my practice, I have rarely seen leg cramps or restless leg syndrome without associated back problems.[22] Proper treatment of the back often relieves the leg problems.

Xylocaine and other local anesthetics reduce pain by numbing tissues. They may be injected or administered as topical creams or patches. In some places, xylocaine is administered in an intravenous drip. This still needs more research.

Ketamine is an anesthetic used to put patients to sleep in operating rooms. Studies are now showing that, in low doses, ketamine may be useful at quieting overactivated microglial cells, which may help neuropathic pain. It can be administered as an intravenous drip or in topical cream.[23]

Dimethyl sulfoxide (DMSO) is a by-product of the lumber industry, and it remains a controversial substance. Claims have been made that it reduces pain, inflammation, and swelling; promotes healing; scavenges for free radicals; and even transports painkillers through the skin. It is also being investigated as a treatment for interstitial cystitis, a rare connective tissue disorder called scleroderma, cancer, antibiotic-resistant bacteria, and brain trauma. In part, it's the wide array of potential uses that makes scientists skeptical about DMSO; we are used to thinking of a drug as having a single, specific action.

DMSO is a solvent and penetrates the skin very easily. Its known side effects are headache and a strong garlic-type odor from the mouth. It is already widely used in veterinary medicine for swollen and injured joints.

Many of the drugs I've described can be combined by pharmacists into custom creams or gels,[24] which can then be applied to painful areas to give comfort and reduce reliance on oral medications. Some medical plans cover them. Many allopathic physicians have never been trained to prescribe these mixtures, but the pharmacists who work with compounding are very helpful and guided me until I could effectively use these to treat pain.

Hormones

We know that our naturally occurring hormones significantly affect pain and vice versa. There is rich literature on the subject. As of yet, however, there is no clearly best way to balance hormones for pain treatment. Many books on integrative medicine offer differing opinions on the best approach, while allopathic medicine, besides checking testosterone levels in men, largely ignores hormone balance in pain patients. The subject is made particularly difficult to study by the thousands of new chemicals and drugs we are constantly exposed to. Nonetheless, there are some reasonable options without risky side effects.

There are two types of artificial hormones — pharmaceutical synthetic and bioidentical. Pharmaceutical synthetic hormones have structures slightly different from our natural ones and so may cause unforeseen side effects. Bioidentical hormones are exact replicas of our natural ones; and while they may still cause side effects, they are always recognized by the body, which already has a system in place to process them. Whenever possible, I recommend bioidentical hormones. Unfortunately, they have not been studied as extensively as the pharmaceutical versions; they cannot be patented and so do not attract from big companies the money needed to support large studies.

Prohormones

Dehydroepiandrosterone (DHEA) is a prohormone, which means it is used by the body to make other hormones. It is the most abundant hormone in the body. Made from cholesterol, it is converted into progesterone, estrogen, and testosterone as needed.[25] We produce our highest levels of DHEA when we are in our twenties, and men have higher levels than women. After our twenties, the levels decrease with age, but the healthiest people tend to have the highest levels in the normal range for their age.[26]

DHEA is connected to the stress system and plays a role in pain and depression. People who are chronically stressed or chronically in pain have low DHEA levels.[27] DHEA, when at healthy levels, modifies our response to stress by blocking the stress hormone cortisol and, as a result, lessening the stress response. Similarly, it may relieve depression by blocking cortisol in the brain.[29] DHEA also changes how pain is transmitted and perceived in the brain, and higher DHEA levels may be associated with faster recovery from pain.[30]

Regular exercise naturally raises DHEA levels. In some cases, to break the cycle of stress and pain, I also recommend DHEA as a supplement. In these instances, I recommend it to patients for three to six months and then wean them off of it. As a supplement, DHEA improves energy and quality of sleep and reduces stress and, often, pain. DHEA supplements should be used only under the supervision of a knowledgeable health care provider.

HORMONES AND NERVE CELLS

Pregnenolone, another prohormone, promotes neurogenesis – the making of new nerve cells in the part of the brain called the hippocampus.[28] The hippocampus is important for memory and pain. Until a decade ago, it was assumed that the adult brain did not make new nerve cells and could not heal itself after the age of twenty-five. We now know this is not the case, and in continuing to study neurogenesis, we may learn interesting ways to reduce pain.

Sex Hormones

While estrogen and progesterone are primarily female hormones, small amounts are also present in men. Estrogen's relationship to pain is confusing. On one hand, it has been shown that estrogen makes females more sensitive to pain — especially during pregnancy.[31] On the other hand, studies show that estrogen can improve pain tolerance.[32] Obviously we don't yet have all the answers.

For optimal health, we need a balance of estrogen and progesterone. If estrogen levels are too high, the result is a condition called estrogen dominance. This causes irregular periods, premenstrual syndrome, breast tenderness and swelling, depression, weight gain, fatigue, insomnia, and more. Estrogen dominance is common in Western societies because of xenoestrogens — artificial chemicals in plastics, cosmetics, and pesticides that act like powerful estrogens once they are in your body. Obesity and diets high in the wrong type of fats also increase estrogen levels in both females and males. In these cases, fat cells act like estrogen factories and convert other hormones, including testosterone, into estrogen. Once you are overweight, estrogen dominance makes it difficult to lose weight.

Women in their perimenopausal years experience a drop in progesterone.[33] This happens ten years before they experience a drop in estrogen and, as a result, women often lack progesterone during these years.[34] These women can balance their hormones by taking bioidentical progesterone — often as a pill or cream. Bioidentical progesterone replacement is generally well tolerated and is not associated with the risks of estrogen replacement, which include blood clots and cancer. This cannot be said of progestin, which is pharmaceutical synthetic progesterone. Progestin is associated with many serious side effects and does not have the same health benefits as natural progesterone.

Estrogen can also be replaced, but this is not necessary for most women. The only exception is a small percentage of women whose hormone imbalances will not improve without a small dose of estrogen in addition to progesterone. I do not recommend taking estrogen without also taking bioidentical progesterone — not even for women who have had a hysterectomy.[35] Occasionally women feel down or depressed from taking progesterone. These women should immediately discontinue the therapy.

Progesterone is now recognized as having a role in improving bone density, sleep, memory, concentration, energy levels, and libido.[36] In addition, animal studies suggest progesterone alters pain by affecting nerves, the spinal cord, and the brain,[37] and it may therefore also prove useful in premenopausal women and in men. Unlike estrogen, it is not feminizing.

Testosterone is primarily a male hormone, but low levels are also present in women. It is an anabolic steroid that preserves bone density and muscle mass. As we get older, testosterone levels naturally decrease, and opioid use can cause deficiencies. Testosterone supplementation is available but controversial, and it is banned for competitive athletes as a performance-enhancing drug. It also comes with significant risks, which include prostate cancer in men. We don't know if it actually causes prostate cancer or just stimulates the growth of cancer cells that are already present. For aging men, however, both options are risky, as older men usually have at least a few cancer cells in their prostate regardless.[38] In most cases, these few cancer cells do not affect the man's health, but extra testosterone may stimulate them to grow into full-blown cancer.

There is lots of interest in testosterone supplementation as a way to improve libido in aging men and women. Except in cases of extreme deficiency, however, the correlation between the hormone and sexual desire is not clear. I have seen patients who have normal levels of testosterone but a poor libido, and others who have low levels of the hormone and an excellent libido.

Growth Hormone

This hormone is controversial in both conventional medicine and complementary and alternative medicine. Antiaging groups promote its use to stimulate muscle bulk,[39] but healthy-aging groups are more wary of it, trying instead to focus on those things that naturally encourage our own growth-hormone secretion. Melatonin and sleep encourage growth-hormone secretion, as does vigorous exercise. If it is used, growth hormone is given as a daily injection.

Cortisol

A stress hormone secreted by the adrenal glands, cortisol is anti-inflammatory. Normally, cortisol levels are high in the morning as you wake and prepare to be active, and low at night as you prepare to rest. When you are overstressed for a long period, this cycle changes. These changes can affect your health and increase your pain.[40]

Abnormal levels of cortisol from chronic physical or psychological stress make you insulin resistant, may play a role in depression and insomnia, and can damage healthy muscle and bone, slow down healing, change metabolism, affect digestion, weaken the immune system,[41] and interfere with the balance of other hormones, including estrogen and testosterone.

As discussed in chapter 5, antidotes to chronic stress include adequate sleep, eating a proper diet, getting regular exercise, and doing daily meditation. There are also some vitamins and herbs that support adrenal function and counteract stress. These are called adaptogens and include vitamin C, rhodiola, ashwagandha, holy basil, and ginseng.

Cortisol levels can be determined by testing blood or saliva samples. Saliva samples, taken four times a day, show changes in cortisol levels and give a more accurate picture of a patient's condition. Blood tests can be inaccurate; a stranger with a needle sometimes causes a patient's body stress, which then releases cortisol beyond normal levels.

Drugs That May Be Causing You More Pain

If you are taking drugs for a medical problem and you also have a pain problem, be aware — the drugs you are taking could be making your pain worse.

Cancer Treatments

There are many different cancer drugs, and they work in a variety of ways. Some are cytotoxic and kill cells, others interfere with the development of new blood vessels needed by tumors to grow, and yet others damage the microtubules that cancer cells use when they multiply. The problem is that each of these mechanisms affects healthy cells as well, including nerve cells. When nerve cells are disturbed, the result may be pain. Chemotherapy cancer drugs can damage nerves and cause pain, numbness, and abnormal sensations called dysesthesias. Radiation therapy is not a drug, but it can still cause pain by damaging normal tissues around the cancer site. Of course, in most cases, the decision to treat cancer should outweigh the possibility of pain. Acupuncture, omega-3 oils, glutamine, and some anticonvulsants and antidepressants have been shown to have a positive impact on pain caused by cancer treatment.

Bisphosphonates

Drugs used to treat low bone density are called bisphosphonates. They can cause bone pain by changing and breaking down the normal internal bone structure. This is most often seen in the jaw and hip, and it usually only happens after five years of taking the drug. This can be a devastating side effect.

Antacids

There are many types of antacids. The simplest ones are the old-fashioned kind, which act to neutralize stomach acid with salts of aluminum, calcium, or magnesium. The effects of these drugs are short-lived and are therefore less likely to cause pain problems. It is, however, best to avoid antacids that contain aluminum — research suggests aluminum might contribute to Alzheimer's disease.

Newer antacids reduce stomach acid by interfering with acid production. The two main drugs that do this are histamine2 receptor antagonists and proton pump inhibitors (PPIs). The most common reason for taking these drugs is GERD, which I discussed in chapter 4. In the case of GERD, these drugs are used to prevent cancer of the esophagus. GERD and cancer, however, is not a simple cause-and-effect scenario; we are prescribing more behind-the-counter antacids than ever before, while the rate of esophageal cancer is growing faster than any other cancer in the United States.[42] In fact, there is no good evidence that these powerful antacids prevent the development of esophageal cancer at all.[43] Some studies even suggest PPIs may be associated with an increase in other cancers, such as cancer of the pancreas.

We don't know the consequences of long-term suppression of stomach acid. The comprehensive review on the website for the American Gastroenterological Association highlights many potential problems and advises caution regarding long-term use.[44] Some of the problems listed have a direct impact on pain, such as by decreasing the absorption of nutrients and heightening the risk of broken bones.

By suppressing stomach acid, antacids can also disturb the balance of the gut's microbiome, which we discussed in chapter 4. Stomach acid is supposed to kill harmful bacteria in our food, and studies show that people on PPIs experience more frequent serious bacterial bowel infections like clostridium difficile and salmonella. In addition, stomach acid is needed to absorb vitamin B_{12}.

There is mounting evidence that people on PPIs and histamine2 receptor antagonists experience more fractures and show signs of inadequate calcium absorption.[45] PPIs now list osteoporosis as a side effect. In addition, the FDA has added a warning to PPIs, saying they can cause a life-threatening deficiency of the mineral magnesium.[46] According to the FDA, magnesium supplements do not improve the problem unless the patient also stops the PPI. Magnesium is needed for the proper functioning of muscles and nerves, and magnesium deficiencies can cause irregular heart rhythms and muscle cramps.

Insufficient stomach acid also reduces the function of a stomach enzyme called pepsin. Pepsin is needed to digest proteins, which provide the building blocks for our muscles, connective tissues, and communication molecules. In general, stomach acid deficiency causes nutrient deficiencies, including those I have mentioned and perhaps others;[47] and nutrient deficiency affects healing, which leaves us vulnerable to pain.

PUTTING YOUR FEET ON THE BRAKES AND THE GAS PEDAL AT THE SAME TIME

When you're on a PPI, your stomach tries very hard to make acid and is geared up to make tons of it as soon as the drug is gone. As a result, if you stop taking a PPI, your heartburn may return. This is called rebound acidity, and it can last for up to two months after stopping the drug. For this reason, I recommend gradually decreasing the dosage of PPIs instead of quitting all at once.

I find that most of my patients are able to discontinue PPIs after changing their diets and habits. I tell the patient to elevate the head of his bed; eat smaller meals; avoid lying down right after meals; reduce alcohol, coffee, and fat intake; quit smoking; and avoid foods that bother him. Taking aloe vera juice and deglycyrrhizinated licorice can also help. If, however, the reflux does not resolve after changing diet and habits, I recommend that the patient continue taking the medication until his heartburn can be addressed in another way by his health care provider.

Cholesterol-Lowering Drugs: Statins

Earlier, we discussed how statins inadvertently affect the body's production of CoQ_{10}. Other negative effects of statins come from their main objective — lowering cholesterol. While statins are commonly used to combat high cholesterol caused by unhealthy food intake, 70 to 80 percent of our cholesterol does not come from food; it's made by our own cells. By interfering with this healthy cholesterol production, statins can cause very harmful side effects. Every cell in our body needs cholesterol, and our nerves and brain are especially dependent on the cholesterol produced by the body — the cholesterol that statins inhibit. There are increasing reports about the harmful effects of statin drugs. These include neuropathy, diabetes, altered production of neurotransmitters, and dysfunction of the energy producers in our cells called mitochondria.[48] All of these are associated with pain.

Rhabdomyolysis is a rare but dangerous muscle complication caused by statins. In the case of rhabdomyolysis, muscle cells leak protein, which causes kidney failure.

Type 2 Diabetes Medications

In recent studies, rosiglitazone has been shown to cause an increase in heart attacks. Metformin causes deficiencies of folic acid and B_{12}, both of which can affect healing and pain. Glyburide has muscle pain associated with it.

Please note: Diabetes is a very serious disease. If you suffer from diabetes, do not take this discussion as a suggestion that you should quit taking your medication. Instead, use this discussion to inspire yourself: use diet, exercise, and stress reduction to control your diabetes, so as to reduce the necessary doses of your medication. Do this only in consultation with your health care providers.

Antibiotics

Fluoroquinolones are a group of antibiotics that have been reported to cause neuropathic pain. This pain can be severe and irreversible. Metronidazole and nitrofurantoin can also do this.

CHAPTER 10

TOXIC STEW

It's an ill bird that fouls its own nest.

— PROVERB

Joanna wakes up to her alarm set right next to her pillow. She gets out of bed and goes to the bathroom. There, she brushes her teeth and takes a shower. In the shower, she cleans herself using body wash, shampoo, and conditioner. She dries herself with her fluffy towel. Then she puts on antiperspirant and her makeup. After leaving the bathroom, she goes to the kitchen, where she makes breakfast. She snacks on cereal while she fries herself an omelet. She eats her omelet on her favorite plate. It turns out that the omelet is too much for her, so she wraps it to take to work.

While this may sound like an ordinary morning, Joanna has actually taken several risks during the first hour of her day. Some people will take exception to the way I refer to the "risks" that Joanna is exposed to. They may say that I am being overcautious, especially when I mention their favorite food additive or convenience product. It is more about the sheer frequency of these exposures than the absolute toxicity of any one, though some of them have long rap sheets.

Joanna's alarm is her smartphone, which she keeps right next to her pillow all night long. She keeps the smartphone's Wi-Fi on, as well. This exposes her to electromagnetic radiation, which has been shown capable of penetrating the skull. Joanna's trip to the bathroom exposes her to fluoride and aspartame, both of which are found in her toothpaste. In the shower, she is exposed to chlorine from the water, and her body wash, shampoo, and conditioner contain parabens, formaldehyde, and hydroquinone. The fluffy towel she uses after her shower has been dried with dryer sheets that contain chloroform, benzyl acetate, pentane, and other toxics. In her antiperspirant, there is aluminum, and in her makeup there are phthalates, more parabens, and lead. Her cereal is made from genetically modified grains that are heavily sprayed with pesticides, and the nonorganic egg in her omelet is from a factory farm where chickens are fed similarly genetically modified grains. Additionally, the hens at the factory farm are inhumanely crowded, and the hens are frequently given antibiotics for the salmonella infection that thrives in those conditions. Her nonstick pan leaches chemicals into the food and the air. In fact, it leaches so many chemicals into the air that, if Joanna had a pet parakeet, the pan's fumes could kill it. Her favorite plate is one of her grandmother's antique dishes, and its glaze contains lead. When she wraps her leftover omelet in plastic wrap, the plastic leaches into her warm food.

Did Joanna really intend to run this toxic gauntlet every morning? Or does she, like most of us, believe that things so commonly used must be perfectly safe?

According to the Environmental Protection Agency, only 7 percent of commonly used chemicals have complete safety data regarding toxicity, and almost half of common chemicals have no safety data at all.[1] Nonetheless, companies are allowed to produce and expose us to these chemicals. Even health or environmental problems associated with a chemical are not enough to keep it from being distributed; and once a chemical is in the marketplace, banning it and containing damage done is an even harder battle. Many studies show exposure to chemicals still commonly used can cause reproductive damage, cancer, and other serious illness.[2] These studies take into account only individual chemicals; almost nothing is known about how these chemicals react in combinations to affect our health. We are a chemistry experiment.

Studies by environmental groups show we all already have toxic chemicals in our bodies. One study examined toxicity in newborn babies by taking blood samples from umbilical cords. The samples were tested for fewer than 400 chemicals, and they detected up to 232 chemicals in the newborns' blood. If each sample had been tested for all 50,000 of the new chemicals introduced between 1979 and 2013, the number would, without doubt, be much greater.[3] Another study, called *Polluted Children, Toxic Nation*, showed that all generations, across all geographic areas of Canada — urban and rural — harbor chemicals in their bodies.[4]

AROUND-THE-WORLD TOXICS

"Every day, the United States produces or imports 42 billion pounds of chemicals, 90% of which are produced using oil, a non-renewable feedstock. Converted to gallons of water, this volume is the equivalent of 623,000 gasoline tanker trucks, each carrying 8,000 gallons. If placed end-to-end, these trucks could stretch from San Francisco to Washington, D.C., and back. Over a year, this line could circle the earth 86 times at the equator."[5]

Toxics, the word now being used for the overall category of harmful chemicals, affect pain by interfering with our metabolism and health.[6] They do this in many ways. Petrochemicals and plastics act like powerful estrogens in our bodies. Heavy metals, like lead and mercury, attach to our cells, replacing the good metals needed to produce energy and detoxify our bodies. Heavy metals are also neurotoxic, meaning they are harmful to our nerves and brain. So are pesticides.[7] As discussed in chapter 9, prescription drugs too can be toxic, and it has been shown that they currently contaminate our water supplies.

Many of these toxics are lipophilic, which means our bodies store them in fat tissues. Sixty percent of our brain is made up of fat, and many of these chemicals can get stored there.[8] Once these chemicals are in fat tissues, they are difficult to get out. Because synthetic chemicals are new, our bodies do not have pathways to eliminate or detoxify most of them. Consequently, our bodies do unpredictable things with these toxics, and some people are especially susceptible. Like canaries in the mineshaft, these people get affected early by toxic exposure.[9] Their symptoms may include pain.

While we still don't know enough about the connection between toxics, illness, and pain, there are things we can do to protect ourselves. First and foremost, avoid exposing yourself and your family to harmful toxics as much as possible by doing adequate research on the products you use. The books and websites in the Resources section at the back of the book will help with this research. It would be much easier to avoid toxics if products were properly labeled, and I urge you to insist on proper labeling whenever possible.[10] Keep in mind that companies respond to financial pressures more than to pleas for social responsibility. In addition, a healthy diet, exercise, and the other healthy habits we covered in chapter 6 will help your body detoxify as much as possible. It is important for all people to protect themselves from toxics, but I believe it is especially important for pain patients, whose energy reserves are already challenged.

YOUR CHOICE

Do you want to clean your baby's room with chemicals that have not been subjected to safety studies? Or do you want to clean your baby's room with chemicals that have to be proven safe before they can be sold in the market?

Toxic Mimics

The body uses the same molecules to serve many different functions. While this system is efficient, it leaves us vulnerable to foreign molecules that mimic natural body molecules; one foreign molecule can interfere with many different functions. For example, parts of our cells called receptors are particularly vulnerable to toxic mimics. Receptors are normally triggered by the body's communication molecules in the form of natural chemicals. The same communication molecule may operate several different receptors all over the body, all of which have very different jobs. If a toxic mimics that communication molecule, it can harm all of the receptors that the molecule operates. When a toxic mimic interferes with hormone balance, the nervous system, the immune system, or the digestive tract, it can cause pain.

FRACTALS

Nature loves to repeat patterns. For example, the pattern of a coastline seen from the sky is the same pattern seen in that coastline's rock fragments under a microscope.[11] So it is with our bodies. Our bodies use the same molecules and patterns to perform different functions.

Heavy Metals

The most common toxic metals in our environment are aluminum, arsenic, beryllium, cadmium, hexavalent chromium, lead, and mercury.[12] Each of these heavy metals is dangerous to our bodies and the environment, and they are made even more dangerous when combined. For example, mercury may be more toxic when aluminum is also present. Both are found in some vaccines.[13]

When heavy metals are in the bloodstream, our body attempts to eliminate them through the detoxification organs — the liver, gut, skin, and kidneys. The body will do all it can to remove heavy metals from the bloodstream; and in the case of high levels, the body will even remove these metals from the blood by storing them in bones and soft tissues. So, just because a blood test shows no signs of heavy metals, this does not mean they are gone from the body — they are just as likely being stored in bones, muscles, fat, hair, the liver, the kidneys, the heart, or the brain. For example, only about 2 percent of lead in adults remains in the blood, while over 90 percent is stored in bones or soft tissues. In children, about 75 percent is stored in the bones. Lead can remain in bones for a lifetime but is often mobilized in the case of pregnancy, breast-feeding, old age, trauma, and broken bones.[14]

Blood and urine tests are most accurate when evaluating a recent exposure to heavy metals — exposure that occurred a few weeks earlier to a few months. When evaluating long-term exposure, biopsies, which are samples taken of body tissues, including fat, muscle, bone, and brain, are more useful. The drawback of biopsies is that they are invasive. Another option is the chelation challenge test. This is done by taking a drug that releases heavy metals from body tissues, after which metal levels can be more accurately evaluated in a urine test.[15]

Lead and mercury are toxic and do not belong in the human body in any amount. Nevertheless, most of us have detectable levels in our bodies from living in polluted environments. In our modern world, lead can be found in old paint, dust, soil, water, and even some children's toys. Mercury can be found in dental amalgams, fluorescent lightbulbs, some thermometers, red tattoo dye, and all fish. In addition, mercury is found in thimerosal, an anti-infective used in some vaccines and other injectable drugs and in medical solutions such as contact lens fluids.[16] Most government health agencies have decided on "normal" levels of lead and mercury in blood and urine tests. It is assumed that, at these normal levels, these metals have no toxic effects. Unfortunately, research suggests otherwise.

Studies show that children exposed to low levels of lead can grow up to have lower intelligence and altered behavior. In fact, studies show an inverse correlation between lead exposure in children and brain development. It seems that children exposed to more lead grow up to have less brain volume. Other studies suggest a relationship between childhood lead exposure and violent behavior.[17] A 2006 study shows that a patient's risk of heart attack and stroke increases in proportion to her level of lead — the higher the lead level, the higher the risk of cardiovascular death.[18] Importantly, this study examined only cases of lead levels within the so-called normal range approved by the US Department of Health. It is also notable that none of the studies mentioned considered cases involving acute lead poisoning, meaning the result of a large toxic dose taken all at once. Additionally, lead has harmful effects on bone healing, normal calcification of our bones, and the function of vitamin D in our bones.[19] There are also concerns that lead causes brain atrophy and cognitive decline in all age groups.[20]

In 2007, a study showed 25 percent of New York City residents had abnormally high levels of mercury.[21] Mercury causes kidney damage, brain and nerve damage, and damage to insulin-producing cells in the pancreas. Mercury levels are also associated with infertility — even when levels are within the normal range.[22] Additionally, a recent study shows that mercury causes increased inflammation.[23]

Mercury can be organic or inorganic. Although inorganic mercury is less toxic, it can be changed into organic mercury in the body by a very common process called methylation. Methylation is not always harmful, however, since it is also responsible for removing mercury from our bodies entirely. The mercury from dental amalgams is inorganic. It stays in our blood for only a very short time but can be stored in tissues for much longer. The mercury in fish is called methylmercury, which is a type of organic mercury. It is also lipophilic, which, as mentioned earlier, means it is likely to be stored in fat tissues. There is genetic variability in our ability to excrete mercury; some people naturally get rid of it faster than others. As a result, some people get sicker at lower doses. Mercury toxicity is also more likely if you also have a zinc deficiency. Chlorella and seaweed can help detoxify mercury, which may explain why the Japanese, who eat fish and seaweed together several times a day, are still in such good health.

LET'S DO SOME MATH

The Environmental Protection Agency regulates the disposal of thimerosal, a mercury-containing preservative used medically. The solution is considered hazardous and requires disposal as a toxin if there is 0.2 mg per liter of mercury. In many flu vaccines there is 25 mcg of mercury in each 0.5 ml dose.[24] This is 250 times more concentrated than what the EPA guidelines define as a toxin. It would be illegal to throw it in the garbage.

SEAWEED AND CHELATION

Wet seaweed wraps are often used in spas and are said to be helpful in detoxifying the body. Studies have identified antioxidants and detoxifiers in seaweeds: organic compounds that attach to heavy metals to remove them from the system.[25] A search of the US National Library of Medicine website shows that there is a growing interest in research on the chelating and other health-enhancing virtues of seaweed.

Lead and mercury are both molecularly similar to calcium and magnesium, which are essential to muscle cells. As a result, lead and mercury may interfere with muscle function, and some studies report muscle weakness, cramping, and pain in people with high levels of lead. Most of these studies examine only acute lead exposures or poisonings and do not evaluate the effects of chronic long-term exposure. In any case, I have often resolved pain in my patients by treating them for heavy metal toxicity.

Tap Water

Studies worldwide have shown that almost every sip of unfiltered tap water contains trace amounts of hundreds of prescription drugs.[26] It seems our water is contaminated by almost every class of drug, including psychiatric drugs, pain drugs, diabetes drugs, blood pressure drugs, statins, antibiotics, anticonvulsants, hormones, and many others. This widespread, constant exposure to drugs is entirely unprecedented. Nobody knows what effect it has on our health, and there are far more ominous questions than available answers. For example, how do these hormones, mostly estrogens, affect our baby boys and girls? Do they affect sexual development? Do they cause premature puberty in girls and do they feminize boys? Do they cause cancers? Do they cause infertility by reducing sperm counts in men and disrupting the normal balance and menstrual cycles in women?

Antibiotics work better on people who have not been exposed to them before, and the effect of constantly consuming antibiotics is unclear. In addition to affecting our bodies when we drink them, antibiotic residues may help evolve drug-resistant "supergerms" like methicillin-resistant *Staphylococcus aureus* and toxic strains of *E. coli*, which are together responsible for almost twenty thousand deaths every year.[27] Similarly, the antiviral Tamiflu has been found in the water supply, and we already have Tamiflu-resistant flu strains.

While I hope most people agree that this long-term, low-dose, involuntary exposure to medications is unhealthy, a large-scale solution is still out of reach. In the meantime, filter your water.

Genetically Modified Organisms

Genetically modified organisms (GMOs) are organisms whose genetic material has been altered by scientists. These organisms are most commonly used to produce genetically modified foods, which are useful to the food industry because they can be cheaper to produce, transport, and preserve. Such foods are also often larger and appear to have fewer flaws. Nonetheless, their downside greatly outweighs their benefits, and GMOs may have unpredictable and unintended effects on consumers. Increasingly, studies are suggesting that GMOs may not be safe. One study shows rats fed on genetically modified corn develop tumors and die prematurely compared to rats fed on a non-GMO food.[28]

It is also becoming more and more difficult to control GMOs, and many non-GMOs, even those in nature, are being contaminated by genetically modified stock. We have already seen genetically modified corn, soy, and papaya pollute natural, non-GMO seed stock. Recently, scientists inserted eel genes into salmon to make them grow twice as fast as normal salmon. Some fish producers want to introduce these salmon into

RISING RATES OF ALLERGY

Seventy percent of our corn, 90 percent of our soy, and 75 percent of our processed food now contains neurotoxins, novel proteins, and allergens. One in every twelve to thirteen American children suffers from food allergies.[29]

fish farms to increase farm productivity. There can be no guarantee that these supersalmon will never escape into the wild, interact with normal salmon, and contaminate wild salmon populations with genetically modified genes.

Over sixty countries require labeling of GMOs, and a growing number of countries are banning them altogether for lack of long-term studies that would assure they are safe as part of the food supply. Currently, GMOs are still legal in the United States, and the FDA does not require any safety studies for them. I personally stay away from genetically modified foods whenever possible. Companies in the United States, however, are not even required to label genetically modified foods as such, making it difficult to completely avoid them.

Electromagnetic Radiation

The technology that allows for worldwide instantaneous communication is nothing short of miraculous. Nevertheless, these new inventions may harm our health. Microwave-emitting devices, which include all cell phones and Wi-Fi systems, constantly bathe us and much of the world in electromagnetic radiation (EMR). When you use a microwave-emitting electronic clicker to close your front gate from fifty feet away, or use your Wi-Fi Internet connection (and are awash in EMR from your neighbors' Internet connections as well), these signals not only penetrate floors, ceilings, and walls but also every living thing in their path.

Originally, scientists believed that EMR could not harm humans so long as it was kept in a range that doesn't heat human tissues. We now know this isn't true. EMR can affect electromagnetic energy, which runs our body's systems; and scientists are now beginning to recognize that even low-energy EMR from electronic devices can negatively affect our bodies. In 2001, Leif G. Salford, MD, PhD, of the Department of Neurosurgery at Lund University in Sweden, said, "The voluntary exposure of the brain to microwaves[, a form of EMR,] from hand-held mobile phones by one-fourth of the world's population has been called the largest human biologic experiment ever."[30]

Several studies have shown that EMR from cell phones can damage the blood-brain barrier, which protects the brain. This can cause leakage of toxic substances into the brain and can affect nerve and glial cells.[31] Some studies also link EMR from cell phones to memory changes and DNA damage. Additionally, there is growing concern that carrying cell phones in pants pockets causes infertility and testicular cancer. Cell phone companies themselves warn in their packaging materials that cell phones should be kept away from the body even when not in use. Of course, people rarely read all the way through this material, and a walk down the street will show you how many people do not follow these guidelines.

Few of us are likely to become totally unplugged; we are too addicted to our gadgets, myself included. We can, however, make some adjustments to reduce our exposure. In the case of cell phones, don't carry your phone on your body, and use a wired headphone whenever possible. At home, give up cordless phones for wired ones. Keep your laptop off your lap, or use a radiation shield under it. Microwave ovens alter the molecules in our food and should be avoided, but if you have to use one, stand very far away while it's on. Some people are more sensitive to EMR than others and experience pain with exposure.

Xenoestrogens and Neurotoxins

Two large classes of toxics, xenoestrogens and neurotoxins, include thousands of individual chemicals, such as parabens, phthalates, and atrazine.[32] Many of these toxics are found in everyday products, including cosmetics, skin care items, cleaners, plastics, foaming agents, flame retardants, petroleum products, pesticides, and many more.

These classes of toxics are of particular concern when it comes to pain. Xenoestrogens and neurotoxins interfere with hormones and nerve cells, respectively. As discussed in previous chapters, proper hormone balance and a healthy nervous system are crucial for healthy, pain-free living.

The Future

I have been a pain doctor for more than twenty years, and in that time I have seen a significant increase in complicated pain syndromes. I suspect that much of this has to do with the increasing toxicity of our everyday lives — the toxic stew we live in. Luckily, health care professionals are beginning to sound the alarm: this toxic load has consequences for our health. Our society is beginning to take notice of the studies showing that fertility rates are declining, cancer rates in children are rising, and every new generation is seeing more chronic disease. The connection between toxics and pain conditions needs to be studied further. In the meantime, we need to stop thinking of these chemicals as "safe until proven unsafe." Our health could hang in the balance.

WE ARE WAITING TO FALL OFF THE CLIFF BEFORE WE INSTALL A GUARDRAIL

Philip J. Landrigan, professor and chairman of preventive medicine at Mount Sinai School of Medicine in New York City, testified about the effects of pesticides before a US Senate committee in 2002, saying, "Pesticides have been shown to cause injury to human health, as well as damage the environment. The health effects include acute and persistent injury to the nervous system, lung damage, injury to the reproductive organs, dysfunction of the immune and endocrine systems, birth defects, and cancer....The notion of the possible 'subclinical toxicity' of pesticides has gained increasing attention in recent years. This term denotes the idea that relatively low-dose exposure to certain chemicals, pesticides among them, may harm various organ systems without producing acute symptoms or being evident in a standard clinical examination. The concept arose from studies of children exposed to relatively low levels of lead who were found to have suffered loss of intelligence and altered behavior even in the absence of clinically detectable symptoms. The underlying premise is that there exists a continuum of toxicity in which clinically apparent effects have asymptomatic, subclinical counterparts. It is important to note that these subclinical changes represent truly harmful outcomes and are not merely homeostatic or physiological 'adjustments' to the presence of pesticides."[33]

PART III

THE NEXT STEPS

CHAPTER II

YOUR TEAM

Alone we can do so little; together we can do so much.

— HELEN KELLER

I have already covered many ways you can begin healing on your own, and part 2 is mainly about helping yourself. I mean this to be empowering, not isolating; you are in control but not alone. There are many professionals, called clinicians, who want to help you. Clinicians include all trained professionals who provide treatment — surgeons and yoga instructors alike. Although they are all professionals and experts in their fields, clinicians should not intimidate you. They work for you, and you should think of them as being on your side — on your team. With their help, you can form new goals and choose a better path toward healing. In this chapter, I suggest different options for therapists, or team members, who can help you.

"Good doctors use both individual clinical expertise and the best available external evidence, and neither alone is enough. Without clinical expertise, practice risks becoming tyrannized by evidence, for even excellent external evidence may be inapplicable to or inappropriate for an individual patient. Without current best evidence, practice risks becoming rapidly out of date, to the detriment of patients."
– David L. Sackett, William M. C. Rosenberg, J. A. Muir Gray, R. Brian Haynes, and W. Scott Richardson, "Evidence Based Medicine"

As mentioned in chapter 2, the 2009 report released by the Office of the Surgeon General mandates integrative pain care as the solution to the problems with the current system of pain care. The report recommends that pain be treated by an interprofessional team, meaning a team made up of professionals from different backgrounds who share information and treatment strategies to achieve the best outcomes for patients. In the ideal future, there will be clinics that incorporate the concept of interprofessional teamwork. For now, there are few settings where this exists; and elsewhere you, the patient, must create your own team. When choosing your team and the treatments they provide, keep in mind there is usually not simply one right answer. For most of us, there are many paths to healing.

The surgeon general's report also recommends a shift in therapeutic order. Whereas the old allopathic order started with drugs, expensive tests, and highly invasive procedures, the new integrative order begins with low-tech, hands-on, low-risk interventions such as chiropractic, acupuncture, and yoga.

Listed here are therapies you may recognize as conventional, and others that fall into the broad category of complementary and alternative medicine. You may come across some you have never heard of before. I include research and plausible explanations for treatments where they exist. Where explanations don't exist, I recommend trusting results. As a scientist, I am interested in how every treatment works. Nevertheless, as a clinician, I am more interested in knowing that a treatment works than in understanding how it works, especially if the risk of causing harm is low.

A Case of Work-Related Injuries

Juan works for a prominent national newspaper. He is the editor of a weekly section and writes special-interest stories. Five journalists report to him. Four years ago, he started to notice pain and stiffness in his wrists. At that time, he would wake some nights with numbness in his hands. About two years ago, he noticed soreness and tightness in his right shoulder, and the numbness in his right hand came more frequently. He also developed a bump on the back of his right wrist and two smaller bumps on the palm side of his fingers — one on the right middle finger and one on the left index finger. The bumps were sore, and he began to literally lose his grip. The two fingers with bumps would sometimes get stuck in the bent position, and it would be painful to straighten them. Once, this caused him to drop a glass of water, and he began to have trouble using scissors.

Difficult financial times led Juan's newspaper to cut staff, including most of Juan's team. Now, he needs to work harder to get his assignments done, and his wife is becoming concerned about him. He constantly wakes at night in pain, his hands look puffy, and he has extreme difficulty moving his right thumb. Juan's wife makes an appointment for him to see his doctor. At the appointment, the doctor prescribes a nerve conduction test and refers him to a surgeon as well. The results of Juan's nerve conduction test are normal. The surgeon checks the bumps on the fronts and backs of his hands and gives them names. She calls the big bump on the back of his right wrist a ganglion, and diagnoses the problem with his index and middle fingers as trigger finger and the problem with his thumb as de Quervain's tenosynovitis. She suggests either steroid injections or surgery.

Juan tells his wife about the visit. He would have to take a lot of time off work for surgery and even more during the rehabilitation period.

This makes him uncomfortable. He considers the injections instead and returns to his family doctor to discuss his options. The doctor has just attended a seminar on repetitive strain injuries, which are work-related injuries commonly affecting the hands. He has heard of some therapies that may work without surgery. The doctor looks up the physical therapist who gave the seminar and sends Juan to see him.

When Juan arrives at the physical therapist's office, he is surprised to see that there are also other practitioners listed on the wall, including a massage therapist, a kinesiologist, a Reiki therapist, a chiropractor, and even a regular MD. The way this clinic works, Juan has to see the doctor first. She takes a detailed history and examines him. She starts by looking at the way he walks and his posture. She then examines how his neck, back, and shoulders move. Juan wonders why the doctor is examining his neck and back when he is there for wrist and hand problems. The doctor explains that the nerves in the hands begin at the neck, and that to understand what is wrong in the hands it is necessary to start at the source. She also explains that posture affects the neck and, as a result, the hands. Posture is the alignment of the different parts of the body.

After her examination, the doctor tells Juan that he hangs his head forward when he leans forward at his computer, which has changed his everyday posture. His shoulders are rounded forward and, as a result, some muscles have shortened. The short muscles are weak, and they sometimes put pressure on the veins, arteries, and nerves that run from his neck to his hands. She shows him that he has a decreased range of motion in his neck and wrists. He has tight and sore muscles in his neck, shoulders, upper back, chest, arms, and forearms.

The proposed steroid injections and surgeries would have addressed only the problems in his hands. The hands, however, are like the tip of the iceberg: they are just the easiest part to see. Chopping off the top of the iceberg will not solve iceberg problems, the doctor explains; operating on Juan's hands would not fix his neck, shoulders, and arms. She explains that there are therapies that treat the root causes, which are his bad posture and tight muscles. Addressing the root causes will also improve the ganglion cyst, the trigger finger, and the de Quervain's.

Juan's treatment plan includes therapies I discuss in this chapter, including Gunn IMS (dry needling), massage, manual therapies, and stretching exercises.

Energy Medicine

Every cell in your body produces and needs energy to function, and we are beginning to see that some pain conditions are caused by deficits in energy production.[1] Although every therapy listed in this chapter affects the energy of the body and could be called an energy therapy, there are also some specific therapies that identify themselves as energy techniques. These include Reiki, qi gong, and acupuncture. While these techniques have been around for thousands of years, scientists are just now developing the technology required to properly study energy medicine. For example, functional MRIs can detect changes in patients undergoing energy therapy treatments, even if the treatments are delivered from a distance.[2]

Cognitive Behavioral Therapy

There are many useful psychological approaches to pain and distress. Cognitive behavioral therapy is one well-researched and effective form of psychological therapy. It helps us reframe automatic negative thoughts that we may have regarding our situation. As I discussed in chapter 5, our thoughts influence our emotions, behaviors, and body chemistry. Cognitive behavioral therapists help us work with the judgmental, inaccurate, and imprecise thoughts that stand in the way of healing.

Myofascial Therapy

The myofascial system is made up of our muscles and the connective tissue, called fascia, that holds us together. Fascia is found everywhere in the body, and myofascial pain syndrome (MFPS) is the commonest cause of pain.[3] Sometimes we develop it as a result of a specific injury. Other times it develops as we go about our day-to-day lives accumulating a series of small injuries. The hallmark of MFPS is tight, shortened muscles with tender areas called trigger points. Our shortened muscles can put pressure on nerves, arteries, and veins. They can also squeeze bones together and cause excess wear and tear on joints. Additionally, these shortened muscles can tug on tendons, causing tendons to be inflamed or thickened. These damaged tendons can develop bumps on them or get stuck in tight places.

MFPS plays a role in pain problems such as low-back pain, neck pain, whiplash, rotator cuff disorders, hip pain, repetitive strain injuries, carpal tunnel syndrome, tennis and golfer's elbow, and trigger finger. It is even involved in many cases of herniated discs, arthritic joints, and migraine headaches.

The tight, shortened muscles caused by MFPS are treatable. In most cases, this treatment at least partially relieves pain. When you lengthen muscles, you reduce the tugging on associated structures. Lengthening the muscles across a joint eases pressure on the joint and reduces wear and tear. Depending on the condition of the joint, some pain may persist, but it usually becomes more manageable. Lengthening muscles also increases their strength; muscles are stronger when they have their full length to generate force.

Myofascial pain responds very well to treatment, and almost every pain problem should be assessed for an MFPS component. Many professionals can assess you for MFPS, including, but not only, osteopaths, chiropractors, physical therapists, massage therapists, and some specially trained allopathic doctors.

Acupuncture

Acupuncture has been around for at least five thousand years and is part of a larger system of medicine called Traditional Chinese Medicine. Treatments entail the use of fine needles to change your flow of energy, called chi, along energy pathways, called meridians, in your body. For a long time, Western medicine has tried to find physical structures that correspond to meridians — structures that carry energy the way arteries carry blood or nerves carry electrical impulses. Although this search has mostly been in vain, some evidence of the existence of meridians has been found on functional MRIs.[4]

Acupuncture can be helpful for many medical conditions, including pain. It relaxes muscles, decreases inflammation, and alters the mediators of stress and pain, including the hormonal system and the parasympathetic and sympathetic nervous systems. When being treated with traditional acupuncture, people often do not feel the needles, which are usually left in place for twenty to thirty minutes. The needles may be heated, turned, or attached to gentle electrical stimulation.

Clinical studies have shown acupuncture can help back pain, osteoarthritis pain, nausea, drug addiction, and more conditions. In 1996, the World Health Organization concluded that acupuncture has been proven to help twenty-eight conditions and shows promise for treating another sixty-three.[5] The National Center of Complementary and Alternative Medicine, a branch of the National Institutes of Health, decided there is substantial evidence that acupuncture is effective and pronounced it acceptable for treating many pain conditions.[6]

BATTLEFIELD ACUPUNCTURE

Ear acupuncture, in a protocol developed by Richard Niemtzow, MD, is being used for pain relief in military settings. This form of acupuncture is being studied for its ability to reduce the use of pain medications and for its ability to give rapid relief in battlefield settings. A similar ear-acupuncture program was developed at Lincoln Hospital in the Bronx to get drug addicts off of drugs.

Dry Needling, Intramuscular Stimulation, and Gunn IMS

Dry needling, as implied by its name, uses needles with no injection. A different name for dry needling is intramuscular stimulation (IMS), which I find more accurate.

IMS uses the same types of needles as acupuncture, but they are not inserted at the traditional acupuncture points, and the practice is not part of Traditional Chinese Medicine. Instead, in IMS, needles are inserted at points determined by Western scientific knowledge of anatomy and physiology. The needles are usually left in place for only a few seconds.

When the needle is inserted, you may feel your muscle release immediately. You may also feel your muscle jump or slowly cramp, then relax. A deep aching is normal. All of these sensations are caused by your muscle lengthening. In most cases, IMS will immediately improve a patient's range of motion. As mentioned earlier, lengthening muscles addresses the root cause of many problems and can reduce pain.

I was trained in a particular form of IMS called Gunn IMS, developed by C. Chan Gunn, MD, and I find Gunn IMS to be the most effective form of IMS. Dr. Gunn developed a theory to explain why people develop shortened muscles and chronic, painful trigger points (TrPs).[7] His theories explain that our spine slowly degenerates as we age, and that there may be changes to our spine very early on, even before X-rays show abnormalities.[8] These early changes, Gunn's theories suggest, put subtle pressure on nerves as they exit the spinal column, which causes muscles to be hypersensitive and leads to short, tightened muscles and TrPs.[9] According to Gunn, an individual's symptoms change depending on the spinal nerves affected, and Gunn has shown that an individual's distribution of TrPs follows the pattern of her affected spinal nerves. Those trained in Gunn IMS insert needles into muscles while following appropriate nerve patterns. These IMS practitioners, myself included, would treat not only Juan's symptomatic muscles in his shoulders and arms but also the muscles close to the affected nerves in his neck, which are closest to the source of his problems. And we would treat signs of shortened muscles farther down Juan's spine, even if he has no detectable symptoms there.

Practitioners of Gunn IMS pay close attention to the muscles close to the spine and nerve roots, while IMS practitioners unfamiliar with Gunn's work usually do not examine or treat the spine as a matter of course. Additionally, Gunn IMS practitioners usually treat more of the muscles than regular IMS practitioners do.

Manual and Stretch Therapies

The therapies listed here are physical treatments used to mobilize and realign different parts of the body or mobilize its energy.

Physical Therapy

Physical therapists (PTs) are experts in rehabilitation. They help you train your muscles to function as efficiently as possible, which is especially important for everyday activities. Painful conditions such as arthritis, broken bones, and myofascial injuries change the way your brain instructs your muscles to do their job. For example, a shoulder injury may change the way your brain coordinates the muscles in your neck, shoulder, arm, and hand to reach for a glass of water. This new coordination is almost certainly less efficient, and it delays the healing process. PTs can help with motor pattern retraining, which speeds up recovery.

PTs are especially good at examining, diagnosing and treating patients after surgeries. They can also treat patients with arthritis and musculoskeletal injuries. These therapists mostly focus on special exercises to rebalance the body, strengthen weakness, and promote function, but some use massage and stretching techniques. Sometimes, but less commonly, PTs are trained in mobilization techniques that improve joint alignment and function. In some countries, acupuncture and IMS can also be done under the title of "physiotherapy or physical therapy." Some PTs use devices such as TENS units, microcurrent devices, or cold lasers.

To be licensed, a physical therapist needs a graduate, master's, or clinical doctorate degree.

Chiropractic

Chiropractic assesses and treats pain and dysfunction by focusing on the alignment of the spine, bones, and joints. Chiropractors often use manual therapies, called manipulations or adjustments, to improve the alignment and motion of these parts.[10] Adjustments can reduce tissue stress and inflammation and encourage healing. Some chiropractors treat muscle tightness with deep-massage techniques called active release therapy and Graston. They may also prescribe exercise for weakness and muscle imbalance. I have found adjustments most helpful when combined with soft-tissue treatments and exercise.

Chiropractors have a four-year postgraduate education, which includes the study of anatomy, physiology, biomechanics, and neurology. In many schools, there is an overall wellness component to chiropractic, and many jurisdictions allow chiropractors to counsel their patients on diet and nutrition. Some chiropractic colleges have developed this wellness component more than others. There are also many postgraduate courses in chiropractic colleges that offer this wellness component, including courses on nutrition, acupuncture and Traditional Chinese Medicine, and homeopathy.

Massage Therapy

Massage therapy can improve circulation in muscles, relieve tight bands and TrPs, and release the abnormally tight fascia that inhibits proper muscle movement. It also helps to release toxics that may be stored in tight muscles. These toxics move into the bloodstream and, from there, are detoxified and excreted. For some people, these toxics cause fatigue and even flulike sensations, including pain and nausea. If you experience this after massage, try drinking a lot of water, taking a bath with Epsom salts, supplementing with extra magnesium, and consuming lots of fiber and detoxifying herbs such as parsley and milk thistle. Those with fibromyalgia often need to begin by being massaged delicately; their condition usually involves tight muscles, toxicity, and a system sensitized to pain.

Some people cannot tolerate deep massage because their systems are too delicate or they are too injured. These individuals can benefit from gentler techniques or a combination of techniques, which might involve gentle soothing massage and deep but very focused TrP work.

You can learn to work on your own TrPs using massage techniques. When doing this, you can use tennis balls, specifically designed balls with bumps on them, or foam rollers. You can also find therapy canes with knobs up and down them, which are useful for reaching TrPs in your own back and neck.

Structural Integration, or Rolfing

Rolfing was the brainchild of Ida Rolf, a doctor of anatomy. It is evident from her writings that Rolf had an understanding of fascia decades ahead of the science of her time. Rolfing involves ten sessions of intense massage-type work meant to reestablish the natural alignment of your body. Some people find Rolfing to be extremely painful. According to Rolf, people experience pain from Rolfing because of their resistance to change, but the process itself is not intrinsically painful.

Osteopathy

In the United States, osteopathic medical schools have the same status as allopathic medical schools, and American doctors of osteopathy can function as full medical doctors. This is not true, however, in other countries, and in Canada osteopaths do not get a medical-equivalent degree. These different educations from country to country make it difficult to generalize about osteopaths. Nonetheless, it can be said that most schools of osteopathy are based on the theories of Andrew Taylor Still, a physician who lived in Kansas in the late 1800s.

The goal of osteopathic treatment, which uses techniques to improve musculoskeletal alignment and vascular and lymphatic regulation, is to enable the body to heal itself. Osteopaths study spinal and joint alignment in great detail, and they use a variety of techniques to help their patients return to optimal alignment. Osteopaths focus on fascia and muscles and use spinal and joint adjustments. They often use a phenomenon called "unwinding" as part of their treatment. Osteopathic theory suggests that our fascia can become tethered or twisted in ways that restrict movement. Unwinding is rhythmic, body-wide movement that releases this tethering. Young babies, as they wake up, have been known to wiggle and writhe, effectively accomplishing the treatment of unwinding on their own. It is suggested that if we could just keep doing these writhing movements all our lives, we might end up with fewer physical symptoms and less pain.

Craniosacral therapy is an osteopathic technique based on work begun by Dr. John Upledger in the mid-1970s. Upledger found that the fluid within the structures of the cranium, the spinal column, and the sacrum has an ebb-and-flow pattern. He showed that if some trauma interferes with this flow, symptoms ensue. This trauma can happen at any time, including as early as birth, and the subsequent symptoms can persist indefinitely until addressed by therapy. Craniosacral therapists use gentle pressure on parts of the craniosacral system to correct abnormalities. I have been treated with craniosacral therapy and have found that the skill with which a good practitioner can feel subtle changes with his hands is remarkable. It is a gentle technique, and it can be tolerated by even very ill and debilitated adults and babies.

Somatoemotional release is a phenomenon introduced to osteopathy by Upledger, who found that stress can cause our muscles do more than just tense up and shorten; it can also cause them to hold on to chemical mediators. Some of these chemical mediators are responsible for our emotions; and if, upon releasing a tense muscle, these mediators are also released, emotions may be experienced. This type of release can occur during a variety of manual therapies, and I have seen it happen as a result of massage techniques and IMS. If you experience this release, you may feel intense emotions that you recognize as being unrelated to your present emotional state. It is common to experience somatoemotional release on tight shoulder and neck muscles because many people carry their stresses in these muscles.

Stretching

I've always been a fan of stretching. It makes people feel good, it helps stimulate circulation in tissues, and it works most of the time. When I was in Canada, I helped develop workplace stretches that reduced pain in my patients who had repetitive strain injuries. Stretching improved these individuals' ability to work and sped up their healing. Stretching always seemed to me like a straightforward mechanical concept: when you stretch a muscle, it lengthens in the direction of the pull. More recently, however, research has shown something unexpected.

The work of Jay Triano, DC, PhD, shows that when a muscle is stretched, only 20 percent of the force of the pull goes in the direction of the stretch.[11] As early as the 1960s, Rolf explained how force is distributed through the web of fascia. If there is a tug in one area, it causes forces to spread in all directions. Imagine tugging at the corner of a wool sweater: the sweater gets distorted in many directions because its fibers intertwine at different angles. While stretching may not be the straightforward mechanical concept I thought it was, this research only further convinces me of its benefits.

Additionally, this new understanding of fascia could account for why certain injuries or surgeries cause symptoms in areas that are not mechanically or neurological connected to the affected area.[12] It is likely that injuries or surgical incisions affect the knit of the sweater — the distribution of forces in the web of fascia.

Stretching can be facilitated by a therapist or done on your own.

Therapeutic Touch

Touch is crucial for our development; babies don't develop properly if they are not touched. Harry Harlow famously showed this in a series of excruciating experiments in which monkeys were raised without touch and became severely disturbed as a result.

Touch calms and balances the parasympathetic and sympathetic nervous systems. For those in pain, touch communicates human connection and is especially important. The simple laying of hands on a patient is one of the most primitive therapies. It has been used throughout human history and is a component of almost every form of therapy.

EARTHING

Our ancestors were literally "in touch" with the earth; they walked, ran, sat, and slept directly on the ground. We, for the most part, are not, which may mean we lose healthy benefits. The earth has an endless supply of electrons that can be used to neutralize free radicals that build up in our bodies. Being in direct contact with the earth through grass, sand, dirt, and even, to some extent, stone and uninsulated concrete allows us to freely use the earth as a source of electrons and reduce oxidative stress. Being grounded on the earth may be very helpful for some people in pain. For more information about the research and about ways to get grounded, refer to the book *Earthing* by Clinton Ober, Stephen Sinatra, and Martin Zucker.[13] I have personally been able to reduce my own pain this way.

In the 1970s, therapeutic touch was developed by Dolores Krieger, a professor of nursing, and Dora Kunz, a natural healer. In therapeutic touch, the therapists' hands hover above or gently touch the person being treated. Most practitioners are nurses. The technique promotes relaxation, pain relief, and perhaps healing in patients. It can be very helpful in hospice and end-of-life work. This is probably the most accepted form of complementary and alternative medicine and energy medicine. It's unclear why this is the case, but it's perhaps because therapeutic touch has been the domain of nurses. Nurses are generally regarded as practical and so may have had an easier time flying beneath the radar of critics of complementary and alternative medicine.

Reiki

Reiki is a system of healing introduced in the early 1900s by Dr. Mikao Usui.[14] It has not been adequately studied. Nevertheless, the National Center for Complementary and Alternative Medicine regards Reiki as safe, and I see no harm in it. In fact, I have seen many patients helped by it.

Practitioners perform Reiki by holding their hands above a patient's body. Reiki treats holistically, affecting the body, emotions, mind, and spirit. Reiki practitioners can feel a sensation as they pass their hands over a patient and may detect disturbances in the energy of the body. Sometimes, these energy disturbances coincide with the symptomatic body parts. Reiki can also be done at a distance, without direct contact between patient and practitioner.

Orthotics, Splints, and Orthopedic Appliances

Splints and casts are essential for some painful conditions like broken bones, torn ligaments, and severe sprains. They can also be useful in other cases, such as carpal tunnel syndrome, de Quervain's tenosynovitis, and extensor and flexor tendinitis. In these cases, splints can easily be overused and should only be used in consultation with your therapist. I usually advise patients suffering from carpal tunnel syndrome to use splints at night to reduce numbness and tingling, but I recommend only intermittent use of splints during the day. For patients with de Quervain's, splints that support the thumb can reduce pain and protect the thumb from excessive movement, but only during the acute phase of the injury. Care should be taken not to become overreliant on splints. They can restrict normal movements and circulation in tissues and can lead to stiffness and even some muscle weakness.

Taping can help support weak ligaments such as ankle sprains and can reinforce proper postures, such as shoulder position. If a splint restricts too much movement or circulation, taping can sometimes be a good alternative. Tape, too, has its disadvantages: it comes off easily and needs special training to properly reapply. I often teach patients to tape their own ankles.[15] There are tons of splinting and taping techniques — enough to fill an entire book.

A heel lift is a small wedge placed under one heel meant to compensate for a difference in leg lengths. We are all slightly asymmetrical; our right side is not the mirror image of our left. Injuries can exaggerate these asymmetries, which can then contribute to pain and delay healing. For many of us, the length of our right leg is different from that of our left, but the difference does not require correction. Seek professional advice to determine if you need a heel lift, how big it should be, and when to stop using it.

Orthotics can be helpful for certain cases of foot, ankle, knee, hip, and back pain. Sometimes the way you walk can cause the rest of your body to make awkward adjustments. Lots of different professionals use different methods to make orthotics. I think the best custom orthotics are made by casting the feet with wet cast materials. Over-the-counter orthotics are all some people need, and they are much less expensive than the custom-made ones.

Physical Medicine Modalities

The following therapies can be supervised by a variety of different professionals. There are other useful therapies as well. Consult your team members for recommendations that would best suit your condition.

Hydrotherapy

Any type of therapy in water is hydrotherapy, from relaxing baths to exercise classes with a PT or trainer. Baths with Epsom salts are accessible for most people. Adding some baking soda helps the body absorb more magnesium from Epsom salts.[16] Aromatic and essential oils can be added to the water to improve circulation and ease muscle tension. Rosemary is good for circulation, and chamomile, lemongrass, and bay essential oils can be soothing for painful conditions.

Photonic Therapy or Cold Laser

Photonic therapy is any therapy that uses light. Cutting lasers are used in surgeries, and cold lasers are used to treat pain and promote healing. Cold lasers use lower energy than surgical cutting lasers, and they do not damage tissues.[17]

I have used different types of cold lasers in my practice for nearly twenty years. The quality of the device is important, and good-quality cold lasers help reduce pain and speed up healing.

Magnet Therapies

Magnets have been used for healing since ancient times, when humans discovered magnetite, a naturally occurring magnetic mineral. These days, many kinds of tests and therapies use electrical, electromagnetic, and magnetic forces. While electromagnetic devices are often safer than drugs and surgery, we need to be mindful that sometimes they can have a negative impact on our bodies' natural energies. Electrical current can severely affect the heart, and strong electromagnetic forces should not be used on pregnant women.

I consider magnetics that don't use electricity completely safe. I have seen pain patients who get relief from these magnets, and others who don't.[18] The magnetic products currently on the market differ in strength, pole orientation, material composition, and other characteristics. I suspect that if magnets could be specifically tailored to an individual's needs, more people would respond to them. I respond well to magnets, and for that I consider myself lucky. Two types of magnets give me significant pain relief and accelerate the healing of my muscular injuries. They also have a moderate effect on my headaches.

Transcutaneous Electrical Nerve Stimulation

One of the most commonly used forms of electrical therapy for pain relief, transcutaneous electrical nerve stimulation (TENS) involves pocket-sized devices that transmit milliamp levels of current through sticky patches called electrodes. These electrodes are attached to the skin over painful areas. While we don't actually know how TENS works, there have been many theories.

For some people, TENS stimulation gives continuous relief. For others, the relief wears off over time as the brain gets used to the stimulation and disregards it as background noise. There are computerized devices that randomly generate TENS signals with different wave characteristics. This can keep the brain sensitive to the signal.

Interferential

This therapy applies two very-high-frequency electrical currents to the skin. Pads are placed so that the electricity spreads along the surface tissues of the painful area. The therapeutic effect is thought to come from the interference pattern of electricity.

Microcurrent

This form of electrical stimulation is called microcurrent because it uses microamp electrical current. The attachment is similar to the TENS pads. Microcurrent has been shown to increase cellular energy. The aim is to get the current to pass through the painful area. You need a knowledgeable professional to instruct you on the proper use.

Cranial Electrical Stimulation

This therapy uses electrical devices attached to the ears or near the head to encourage relaxation. The devices conduct microcurrent or TENS milliamp current. Research indicates that patients treated with cranial electrical stimulation have improved mood and sleep and less anxiety. For many, it offers drug-free pain relief. Some of the devices are approved for use in the US Veterans Administration hospitals.

Neuromuscular Electrical Stimulation

This type of electrical stimulation causes contractions in muscles, which strengthens them or improves their function after stroke or injury. Although there is no strong research supporting this therapy, it is safe and may be helpful in individual cases.

Ultrasound

Ultrasound uses sound waves to stimulate injured muscles and tendons. It can increase circulation in the areas treated. Some evidence suggests this therapy improves injuries, but this evidence is not very strong. Ultrasound is used extensively in many physical therapy and chiropractic offices. In my experience, it is one of the less effective therapies. Nonetheless, every once in a while it produces a great result.

GOOD USE OF YOUR TIME AND RESOURCES

When you are getting therapy, make sure you use your time with your therapist well. For example, if you are having ultrasound therapy and are not seeing results, ask your therapist to change to more hands-on therapies. In addition, don't use your time with your therapist for things you could do at home. You can always put on heat or cold packs after the therapy session, so use your time with the therapist for more personalized protocols. Remember, either you or your insurance company is paying for the treatment, so make sure you get good value.

High-Intensity Ultrasound, or Shock Wave Therapy

Shock wave therapy stimulates chronically injured tissues by bombarding them with high-intensity sound waves. This results in small areas of injury and inflammation, which the body then heals. The theory behind this therapy suggests that, as the body heals these new injuries, it also heals the chronic ones. It can be used on chronic tendinitis and calcium deposits in tendons and fascia. The technology is still in development, and it may yet become more effective.

Invasive Procedures

I have left invasive procedures to the end of the discussion because that is where they belong. For chronic conditions, noninvasive therapies should be thoroughly explored before using invasive measures.

Injections

There are many different substances that can be injected in many different structures in the body. I present a few here, along with some details on current evidence of how well they work.

TRIGGER POINT INJECTIONS

Some doctors treat TrPs with injections. These injections are usually local anesthetics but can also contain corticosteroids, vitamin B_{12}, or a homeopathic remedy. When this technique works, it gives patients pain relief that outlasts the few hours of numbness expected from the local anesthetic. We don't really know why TrP injections work. One theory supposes that the local anesthetic interrupts pain pathways temporarily, causing the brain to "forget" about a specific pain for a while. There are, however, studies that show a needle itself may have the same effect without any injection.[19]

Studies do not support the use of corticosteroids for TrP injections,[20] and I prefer not to inject any steroids into muscles and tendons. I have seen many complications from steroid injections and do not recommend them for most chronic pain cases.

INJECTION OF SCARS

Sometimes people have pain around or radiating away from scars. I have worked with patients who have described burning, numbness, pins and needles, sharp pain, dull pain, and other sensations. A series of simple and safe injections into a scar along its full length can sometimes give great relief that is long lasting. I usually inject local anesthetic alone or in combination with vitamin B_{12}. "Neural therapy," which incorporates scar injections, was developed in the 1920s in Germany. I have seen good results in my patients but I have not seen studies done on it.

BOTULINUM TOXIN INJECTIONS

Botulinum toxin can be injected into muscles to weaken or paralyze them. It works by blocking signals between nerves and muscles. The effects last up to three months, and muscles that are repeatedly injected become progressively weaker. This is useful when the improvement in function outweighs the potential side effects of weakness.

The injections can be helpful for treating spasms, headaches, stroke, and cerebral palsy,[21] and they can give relief to migraine patients as part of their treatment. Botulinum toxin is also used to treat dystonia, a movement disorder that causes muscles to contract involuntarily. Like most drugs, it can relieve symptoms but does not address underlying causes. Allergic responses can also develop at any time.

DIAGNOSTIC BLOCKS

Diagnostic blocks are local anesthetics injected around nerves or into joints, used to determine which structures are causing pain. If a diagnostic block significantly reduces pain, a more permanent pain procedure can be considered. The more permanent procedure may involve cutting nerves or deadening them in other ways. To be certain of the result of a diagnostic block, several blocks should be done at different times, and a placebo should be substituted for some of them. A procedure to cut nerves or damage nerve cells should never be done without excellent results from diagnostic blocks.

SPINAL INJECTIONS

These are injections, usually of steroids, to reduce inflammation around an intervertebral disc or a spinal nerve root. Spinal injections can be helpful if the target is carefully chosen and the injection is done with ultrasound or X-ray guidance. The duration of relief varies from patient to patient.

VISCOSUPPLEMENTATION

This therapy entails injecting into a joint a substance that cushions the joint and creates a separation between the bones. This can help cases of arthritis where cartilage has been significantly worn down. Most viscosupplementation products mimic normal joint fluid. The injections are not known to cause any joint damage and may delay the need for joint replacement surgery.

STEROID JOINT INJECTIONS

Steroids are sometimes injected into joints to decrease inflammation. Unfortunately, steroids can also cause the cartilage in joints to deteriorate faster; it's a trade-off. In the case of rheumatoid arthritis, inflammation rapidly damages the joint, and it is worth using steroid injections. In the case of osteoarthritis, there is little destructive inflammation, and steroid injections may cause more harm than relief.

OZONE INJECTIONS

Ozone is a form of oxygen administered by injection. It is used to increase oxygen in joints and tissues. Although ozone is not yet a mainstream therapy in the United States, it is used commonly in Italy, Germany, and other countries. Its effectiveness is well supported by literature, but more research is needed.[22]

Regenerative Injection Therapy

Many in the medical community are interested in finding ways to get parts of the body to repair and regenerate themselves. US military medicine is researching this area extensively. Some of the practices below have been used safely for decades.

PROLOTHERAPY

This therapy injects dextrose and water or other combinations of substances into tendons, ligaments, or fascia. The injection causes mild inflammation and the release of growth factors that stimulate healing. Those with loose joints, stretched or torn tendons, or damaged ligaments respond well to this technique. It restores stability to joints and strength to ligaments and tendons.[23]

PLATELET-RICH PLASMA

Individuals with damaged tendons, muscles, ligaments, or joints can benefit from injections of platelet-rich plasma — blood with a high concentration of platelets, stem cells, and growth factors. The plasma is produced by removing blood from a patient's arm, processing it, usually in a centrifuge, and then reinjecting it into that patient's damaged structures. In theory, the stem cells in it accelerate healing. The therapy gives some people relief and speeds the repair of tissues. It may even rebuild the cartilage in joints.[24]

There is currently no standard for the preparation of platelet-rich plasma. There are many technologies available but inadequate research to fairly compare them.

The Future of Regenerative Therapies

Prolotherapy and platelet-rich plasma are examples of regenerative therapies currently in use. Regenerative therapies — therapies that help tissues regenerate and repair themselves — are the way of the future. Regenerative medicine will one day make many of our current therapies obsolete, and scientists are currently developing therapies that use stem cells to provide us with new intervertebral discs and cartilage for our joints. These therapies retrieve stem cells from inside of us and use them to grow new tissues.

Other Procedures for Pain

The following procedures are more invasive ways of dealing with pain.

Rhizotomies, Radiofrequency Facet Denervation, Cryoablation, Sympathectomies

These techniques affect pain by burning, freezing, or cutting nerves. When you sever the nerve, it usually regrows; and although these procedures may work for a while, if pain returns, it is often harder to treat. Do not undergo any procedure to destroy a nerve before having a diagnostic block, and only consider these procedures if the result of the block is at least an 80 percent reduction in pain. The procedures work best when there is a clear source of pain, and they rarely have positive results when there is no clear cause or in cases of chronic neuropathic pain.[25]

Implantable Devices

Spinal cord stimulators and implantable nerve stimulators are devices that can be implanted around the spinal cord or nerves to block pain transmission. This can be useful in cases where many other forms of treatment have been unsuccessful. These procedures are extremely invasive, and any time a foreign device is implanted into your body there is a chance of infection. Before having this procedure, have a clear discussion with the specialist doing the procedure about how it can help. Make sure to discuss, in detail, the alternatives and risks involved.

Surgery

This section is about chronic injuries. Acute injuries should be assessed by your health care team on a case-by-case basis.

Surgery is sometimes considered as a treatment for painful conditions. Unfortunately, surgery itself sometimes causes pain.[26] John Loeser, MD, puts it well: "During the last three decades, increased data on surgical outcomes have led to the realization that most chronic pain patients do not respond adequately to surgical procedures."[27]

Sometimes exercise and therapy seem like too much trouble, and the "quick fix" of surgery appears easier. What many patients do not realize is that after surgery they will require intensive therapy. If the same level of therapy had been done before surgery, many patients may have improved enough to make surgery unnecessary.

Lumbosacral spinal surgery, which is surgery for chronic low-back pain, is fairly commonplace, accounting for over two hundred thousand surgeries each year in the United States. In some communities, back surgeries get done ten times more often than in other communities. It is often difficult to understand why the surgery rate varies so much when the rate of back problems is fairly steady. In any case, most surgery for chronic low-back pain is unhelpful, and 20 to 40 percent of these patients are left with severe chronic pain.[28] Unsuccessful back surgeries are so common that we have created a name for the result: "the failed back." The name seems to imply the unsuccessful operation is the back's fault.

BACK SURGERY

- Weight loss will help back pain significantly, especially if a patient has too much fat around the belly.
- Graduated exercise, which means gradually increasing the effort needed to do an exercise, is important.
- Microdisc surgery is done through a tiny incision using an arthroscope, an instrument that allows the interior of a joint to be viewed. This type of surgery is preferable, because it causes less tissue damage than regular surgery.

Sometimes carefully done disc surgery relieves pain, but surgery should be done only after a trial of conservative therapy. The conservative therapy may be directed by a PT, chiropractor, osteopath, pain doctor, or physiatrist and should continue for three to six months or longer, unless there are danger signs. These signs include loss of bladder or bowel function or progressive weakness in the limbs. I often see patients who could have avoided surgery had they had a proper trial of conservative therapy.

HERNIATED DISC FALSE ALARMS

If you have back pain and an MRI shows disc abnormality, it doesn't always mean the disc is the cause of the pain. MRIs are so sensitive that they find herniated discs in people who have no symptoms. Time and a well-trained professional are the best ways to figure out if you actually have a troublesome disc. Regardless, the best course for a herniated disc is almost always the natural course, which means letting it improve on its own over time.

Spinal fusion surgery is almost always a revolving-door affair. Surgeons often warn patients that there will be accelerated wear and tear above and below the fusion, and once one spinal segment is fused, a patient will likely have to repeat the surgery for other segments. In certain cases, conservative therapy does not work and fusion surgery is worth the potential drawbacks.

The following conditions do better without surgery, and most of them should never be operated on: chronic repetitive strain injuries like most cases of carpal tunnel syndrome, de Quervain's tenosynovitis, trigger finger, ganglion cysts, extensor tendinitis, and rotator cuff injuries. Carpal tunnel syndrome warrants surgery in the case of a crush injury, severe arthritis, or other disease-causing bony impingement. Sometimes rotator cuff tears and extremely lax shoulders need surgery. In most other cases, working with competent rehabilitation techniques can relieve pain and improve function better than surgery. Modern science has shown us that tissues, even cartilage — which was once thought to be incapable of repair — have the ability to heal themselves.

Joint arthroscopies are surgical procedures in which an arthroscope is inserted into the joint for both diagnosis and treatment. In general, they can be very useful techniques, and they do minimal tissue damage to joints in both acute and chronic injuries. Keep in mind, however, that there is still some tissue damage done by arthroscopes.

My advice is to take good care of your joints and discs. Hopefully, the new regenerative technologies will help us create our own spare parts and, in doing so, avoid many surgeries.

CHAPTER 12

THE ROAD TO RECOVERY

If you don't know where you are going,
you might wind up someplace else.

— YOGI BERRA

Here you are, on your healing journey. Your goal is to improve your function and your health, and you can now take charge with self-care techniques. The integrative approach discussed in this book gives you tools to use even if the exact cause of your pain is still unclear.

In modern medicine, we have become conditioned to expect the big, immediate changes that come from drugs and surgery. As I explained early on, these immediate changes rarely fix very much in the long run. Most true improvements that occur, especially in chronic conditions, come from the slow and natural process of regeneration and repair that is hardwired into us. When you look at it this way, you see that a large part of recovery is the search for the impediments to healing — detective work. Many forces affect healing, and people lead complicated lives, so the road to recovery is neither straight nor the same for everyone. For most people, the road winds and curves. It may feel as if you aren't always moving forward, but don't worry too much about short-term fluctuations in your progress. Remember, worry causes inflammation and a "go with the flow" attitude is healthiest.

If you have chronic pain, you should not let pain be your guide. It can lead you astray and dominate your life. Sometimes pain in the short run achieves relief in the long run, and hurt does not necessarily mean harm. For example, as I mentioned in chapter 8, an exercise program is important for everyone, but it comes with the healthy pain of reconditioning. A professional such as a private trainer, chiropractor, osteopath, or exercise therapist, or a combination of these, should help you determine your safe levels of exercise.

Your body begins life with optimal function. For example, early in life, you start off using the most appropriate muscles for bending over or maintaining posture in your neck. As you get injured, some muscles get overworked or damaged and your body compensates by using different, less appropriate muscles. Over time, compensation patterns may occur. Your body may go through several compensation patterns before it has no more tricks to try. At that point, pain, weakness, and other symptoms develop. Think of all these compensation patterns as a large ball of multi-colored yarn, where each compensation pattern is its own color. Healthy treatment will unravel the ball, but as it does, you will experience each color and the symptoms that come with it. These symptoms may include soreness in particular muscle groups. You may also recognize many of the colors as they unravel; they are compensation patterns you experienced while your body was becoming injured in the first place. As you are working through your therapies and exercise program, it may feel as if your pain is moving. This is a good thing. It means your body is getting closer and closer to the optimal function it began with.

Keep in mind that some injuries will heal completely and some simply won't. In these cases, an individual injury might always need higher maintenance activities, usually in the form of exercise or intermittent care from a member of your treatment team.

In chapter 2, I discussed changing the conversation on pain relief. I

Simon is thirty-two. He has had back surgery to ease pressure on a nerve caused by a herniated disc, which has been accompanied by pain in his back and down his left thigh. It showed up on the MRI, and he was in surgery two weeks later, even though he had none of the danger signs that dictate early surgery and had had no trial of physical therapy for six to twelve weeks first. He was in as much pain after the surgery as he had been before, even though he was told the surgery was a success. Six months of physical therapy after surgery did not help. He was on opioids and could not work. He was offered a second surgery to fuse the joints in the area of his previous surgery — the point on his spine designated as L4-5 — and he decided to do it. He was again told the surgery was a success. Therapy after that surgery brought some relief, but coming off opioids proved challenging.

A year after the fusion, Simon fell on ice and twisted his back, causing pain higher up in his back and in his hips. Another course of therapy did not help, so he went for a series of facet-joint injections done under fluoroscopic guidance. He had the maximum number allowed by his insurance and then was told they could do nothing more for him. He was offered another surgery by his original surgeon, to fuse a level or two above L4-5.

Simon decides to get a second opinion. He goes to see a chiropractor who works closely with both a massage therapist and a physical therapist who does acupuncture. They present him with a plan for therapy to treat the tight muscles in his back and hips and help correct his posture. They set up a treatment schedule and give him a home exercise program. After six months, Simon feels stronger, has less pain, has stopped his daily use of opioids, and is pleased that he did not go for another surgery. He still feels intermittent pain just above the level of his previous surgery.

At this point he visits a physician who uses regenerative therapies. This doctor determines there is too much movement between the small joints called facets that are at the back of the spine. This affects the area above Simon's surgery and is very common. The doctor injects platelet-rich plasma and prolotherapy, to give Simon's back more stability. Simon is very pleased with the results. Now whenever Simon's back "acts up," he gets more serious about his exercise.

talked about reshingling the roof instead of replastering the ceilings. In the following section are questions you can ask in order to change the conversation.

What Should You Do as a Patient
to Keep Your Own Case Organized?

It is important for you to take ownership of your condition and your overall health. Your treatment team is there to provide information and inspiration, but you are the one who has to do what needs to be done to heal.

Answer the first set of questions below for yourself to make sure you understand the assessment process that has led to your diagnosis. The three sets of questions after that are meant to guide your conversations with your treatment team.

The Detective and the Diagnosis

- Did this assessment seem complete? Did it cover all your concerns, complaints, and symptoms? Remember that special tests like MRIs are not the gold standard that we wish they were, and sometimes a careful physical examination tells us more than the test.
- What is the diagnosis? If you don't understand the words used, ask what they mean. Remember, a diagnosis is just a label.
- If the diagnosis confuses you, ask why it is the label being given.
- Are there tests that confirm the diagnosis? How reliable are they?
- Were alternative diagnoses considered by the health care professional? If so, what were they? Are they still being listed as possibilities?

Questions for Your Treatment Team

- How can I best help myself improve? What should I do for myself?
- What do you think is the underlying problem?

- Is the treatment meant to address the symptoms, the underlying problem, or both? (Ask your team this question if they suggest a treatment.)
- How does the treatment work to help the underlying problem and/or the symptoms?
- How will you and I know if it is working? What are the goals and targets?
- How will you adjust the therapy if I do not see progress?
- How long should I wait before I can expect to see some positive changes?
- How do you decide that a treatment isn't working?
- If the first plan does not work well, do you have a plan B?
- How long will it take for me to get better? (This last question is always difficult to answer. I usually say my crystal ball is out at the cleaners, but I respect the patient's right to ask. When I am working with the intramuscular stimulation technique, I tell most patients to expect to see a positive result by the fourth session. Ninety percent of my IMS patients experience a positive result within this time frame. Most other forms of therapy, however, require more sessions before the initial effect is apparent.)

Drug-Taking Etiquette: Questions Every Patient Should Ask

- How can I best help myself to improve? What should I do for myself?
- How do you spell the name of the drug?
- What am I taking the drug for? Which symptoms does it help? Is it actually curing something I have?
- How do I take the drug? What is the starting dose? Do I need to periodically change the dose? When do I take the drug? With meals? On an empty stomach? At bedtime?
- Does this drug interact with other medications, herbs, nutrients, or food and beverages?

- What effects should I expect? Are there any side effects? How quickly do they occur?
- How long will I stay on the drug if it does not seem to be working?
- How long will I stay on the drug if it is working?
- Do you expect me to be on this drug for the rest of my life? If yes, why?
- Has a research study tested this drug to find out if it is safe to take for that long? How long did the study last?
- How long has the drug been on the market, and was it studied specifically for use for the type of problem I have? Is it approved for the problem I have, or is this an off-label use (meaning not officially approved)?
- If the drugs are opioids (which are known to become less effective over time), do you have a plan for when the opioid becomes ineffective?

Questions to Ask When Consulting a Surgeon

- How can I best help myself improve? What should I do for myself?
- What specific symptoms is the surgery going to address? Is it for relief of symptoms, or does it actually correct a problem?
- How long should I try therapy before having surgery? (For most nonemergency situations, this time frame should be three to six months. If your surgeon does not make this recommendation, ask why.)
- How long is rehab after surgery?
- What are the chances that my function will return? How much function will return?
- What are the chances that my pain will be relieved? How much of my pain will be relieved?

Sanjiv had severe pain in the lower abdomen, which doctors had trouble diagnosing. He continued to get worse, and they finally did surgery and found the problem: his appendix had ruptured. The rupture had caused a lot of irritation, and infection had spread internally. They did what was necessary to clean up the area, removed the appendix, and assumed that he would recover.

Sanjiv did well for five years, until he began to develop pains in his abdomen that made it uncomfortable for him to reach overhead or twist his body. He did not seek treatment. Now, fifteen years later, he has developed chronic headaches and upper-back pain in addition to the abdominal discomfort. After going to headache doctors, he is finally referred to an osteopath, who notices that Sanjiv's head is tilted to the left all the time. When seen in profile his muscles seem to be extremely tight, and he cannot take a deep breath to expand his rib cage. The scarring of the connective tissues that started with the burst appendix has progressively restricted the movements of some of his fascia and muscles. Sanjiv's changed posture is the cause of his pain.

Sanjiv works with the osteopath, who brings about fascial releases deep inside his abdomen. He also undergoes Gunn IMS to get releases of the neck and back, because over time these muscles have developed their own injuries from struggling to keep Sanjiv upright. He begins to take yoga classes and to practice at home daily. As his posture improves, his pain resolves.

- What are the chances that I will need another operation in a few years?
- What are the consequences if I choose not to have surgery? Would there be changes in strength, movement, and sensation in the long or short term?
- What are the possible risks or side effects specific to this procedure?
- What is the infection rate at the hospital where I'm having

this surgery? (Statistics for postoperative infections can vary tremendously between institutions, and you want to minimize your risk of serious complications.)

- What defines success for the type of surgery you are planning? (For example, a common definition of success for back surgery for discs or fusions is eighteen pain-free months. Some patients are shocked when they learn this only after their pain has returned. They might not have consented to the surgery in the first place had they understood this limited definition of success.)

Take notes during your visit, or bring a friend who will do that for you. Go home and read the notes. Also read about the procedures and what others have said about their experiences.

Do not let yourself be rushed by external factors, such as the doctor's schedule or the timing of Christmas. Take time to decide if this surgery is right for you.

Most medical professionals will admit that surgery changes things; a back that has never been operated on often does better in the long run than one that has.

Getting Started with Your Own To-Do List

You may have noticed that most of the lists above started with the questions "How can I best help myself improve? What should I do for myself?" Only you have the ability to affect your health twenty-four hours a day, every day, with the choices you make.

- Eat an anti-inflammatory diet, which means eating low-glycemic foods and good-quality proteins, avoiding chemicals in food, and drinking plenty of fresh water.
- Take anti-inflammatory supplements.
- Exercise regularly to the best of your current ability, and expect to improve.

- Identify your sources of stress and try to spend some time de-stressing.
- Take responsibility for getting well.
- Find joy and meaning in your life.
- Find a primary-care practitioner and a treatment team you like working with.

After I gave a talk on the treatment of chronic pain to the trainees at the Arizona Center for Integrative Medicine,[1] one of the students paid me what I regard as a very meaningful compliment. This was the first time she had heard a talk on chronic pain that was not depressing. Talks on chronic pain are often focused on the chronicity of the pain and the difficulties of achieving improvements. This is because the medical community often does not have an optimal repertoire for treating it: the field is dominated by the use of drugs, high-tech testing that is not informative, and high-tech procedures and surgeries that are only sometimes helpful. The talk I gave pointed out other options for diagnosis and treatment — the ones outlined in this book — and gave case studies of people whose pain decreased and health improved.

I hope this book leaves you with both optimism and a long to-do list. In it, I have offered different ways of looking for answers and a more comprehensive set of tools for treating chronic pain than is commonly found — and most of these tools are as simple as choosing healthier options in your life. Remember, a healthy body means less pain. You are much more than just your pain.

ACKNOWLEDGMENTS

Holistic Pain Relief has been a pleasure to write. It brought together several things in my life for which I am grateful: my love of writing, science, and teaching, and the practice of medicine that brings me the great satisfaction of working with my patients, who have taught me ever so many medical and life lessons by sharing their journeys with me. No work of this sort is done without a great debt to others. I gratefully acknowledge the clinicians who went before me and from whose methods I learned. My education in integrative medicine began with an interest in myofascial pain. I had the privilege of learning from Dr. C. Chan Gunn, who has been my mentor since 1991, when I was first introduced to his work through the Acupuncture Foundation of Canada. I was also taught by Drs. Janet Travell and Robert Gerwin.

In my clinical practice, I have been blessed to work with wonderful professionals who have shared their knowledge and skills. My team in Toronto included Mark Gilbert, Dwayne van Eerd, Mary Naumovsky, Lois Singer, Margaret Ranger, Tiziana Schiafone, Denis Marier, Michelle Katz, Andrew Appel, and Linda Finn. I also thank Lisa Dunn, Sharon Foley, and Nancy Winton, who helped keep the office organized; their efforts were invaluable.

This book would not have been written without Seth Gilbert, a talented editor. He edits with care and precision and assisted me in defining the key concepts I have tried to convey. I am grateful to Georgia Hughes, editorial director at New World Library, and her team, including copyeditor Bonita Hurd and managing editor Kristen Cashman, for shepherding the book to its finished form. My agent, Claire Gerus, shared my vision and made the perfect match between the book and New World Library. Malcolm Lester, publishing consultant, encouraged me early on, and I owe him thanks.

I had the help of thorough and enthusiastic research assistants, including Olivia Seibendik, Emma Cashman, Noah Gilbert, Meredith Keller, and Cristina Bemans.

I also thank those who read the early and revised versions of my chapters and offered their much-needed advice. They are experts in their fields, and they include Nora Shulman, Jane Ballantyne, John Loeser, Audrey and Eric Schoomaker, Ping Ho, Randy Horowitz, Steven Devries, Ted Price, Michael Brown, David Rubin, Aviad Haramati, Giana Angelo, Jay Triano, Nancy Harazduk, Felix Tyndel, Joanne Oates, Carolyn Wessels, Carrie and John Greschner, Dawna Treibicz, Rebecca Dale, Judy Turner, Cheryl Ritenbaugh, Steve Lawson, Irakli Soulakvelidze, David Tauben, and Alex Cahana.

Several other experts generously shared their knowledge in interviews, including David Reisman, Russell Jaffe, Jennifer Sass, Bill Martz, and Gareth Owen.

Thanks to all of you for sharing your time and wisdom.

ENDNOTES

Chapter 1. Pain, Nature's Wake-Up Call

1. I am not recommending that people untrained in acupuncture treat themselves with needles. My instructors made sure I knew the safe areas I could treat.

2. S. A. Skootsky, B. Jaeger, and R. K. Oye, "Prevalence of Myofascial Pain in General Internal Medicine Practice," *Western Journal of Medicine* 151, no. 2 (1989): 157–60. (Skootsky, Jaeger, and Oye found that 30 percent of regular patients in a general medical clinic met criteria for MFPS.) S. Marklund and A. Wänman, "Incidence and Prevalence of Myofascial Pain in the Jaw-Face Region: A One-Year Prospective Study on Dental Students," *Acta Odontologica Scandinavica* 66, no. 2 (2008): 113–21. (Marklund and Wänman found that 19 percent of normal dental students develop MFPS over a year.) S. Roach et al., "Prevalence of Myofascial Trigger Points in the Hip in Patellofemoral Pain," *Archives of Physical Medicine and Rehabilitation* 94, no. 3 (2013): 522–26. (Roach et al. found that approximately 90 percent of patients with patellofemoral pain had MF trigger points, and 30 percent of normal controls did.) David G. Simons, "Clinical and Etiological Update of Myofascial Pain from Trigger Points," *Journal of Musculoskeletal Pain* 4, no. 1–2 (1996): 1–2. (According to Simons, between 30 and 93 percent of patients with pain anywhere in the body had myofascial trigger points.)

3. There is, however, a small and unfortunate group of people who have congenital insensitivity to pain, and they are even worse off than the rest of us. Because such a person feels no pain, she may burn herself, bite off her own tongue, or continue to use a limb with a broken bone.

4. Institute of Medicine of the National Academies, *Relieving Pain in America: A Blueprint for Transforming Prevention, Care, Education, and Research* (Washington, DC: National Academies Press, 2011). This report was written by the IOM's Committee on Advancing Pain Research, Care, and Education.

5. Harald Breivik quoted in "World Health Organization Supports Global Effort to Relieve Chronic Pain," October 11, 2004, World Health Organization website, www.who.int/mediacentre/news/releases/2004/pr70/en/, accessed June 1, 2012.

6. Institute of Medicine of the National Academies, *Relieving Pain in America*, 1.

7. A. B. Krueger and A. A. Stone, "Assessment of Pain: A Community-Based Diary Survey in the USA," *Lancet* 371, no. 9623 (2008): 1519–25.

8. Alyssa Brown, "Chronic Pain Rates Shoot Up until Americans Reach Late 50s," Gallup Wellbeing, April 27, 2012, www.gallup.com/poll/154169/chronic-pain -rates-shoot-until-americans-reach-late-50s.aspx, accessed June 1, 2013.

9. Jeffrey Rome, *Mayo Clinic on Chronic Pain* (Rochester, MN: Mayo Clinic, 2002), 2.

10. Andrew Gottschalk and Susan A. Flocke, "Time Spent in Face-to-Face Patient Care and Work outside the Examination Room," *Annals of Family Medicine* 3, no. 6 (2005): 491.

11. H. Beckman and R. Frankel, "The Effect of Physician Behavior on the Collection of Data," *Annals of Internal Medicine* 101, no. 5 (November 1984): 692–96.

Chapter 2. The Changing Times

1. Central Intelligence Agency, "The World Factbook: Country Comparison — Life Expectancy at Birth," undated, https://www.cia.gov/library/publications /the-world-factbook/rankorder/2102rank.html, accessed December 25, 2012.

2. Barbara Starfield, "Is U.S. Health Really the Best in the World?," *Journal of the American Medical Association* 284, no. 4 (2000): 483–85. Dr. Starfield herself died from the side effects of a medication two years ago.

3. Poor diet and physical inactivity account for four hundred thousand deaths, or 16.6 percent of total deaths, per year in the United States (Ali H. Mokdad et al., "Actual Causes of Death in the United States, 2000," *Journal of the American Medical Association* 291, no. 10 [2004]: 1238–45). Based on data collected by the Centers for Disease Control, during 2000–2004 an estimated 443,000 persons in the United States died prematurely each year as a result of smoking or exposure to secondhand smoke ("Smoking-Attributable Mortality, Years of Potential Life Lost, and Productivity Losses — United States, 2000–2004," *Morbidity and Mortality Weekly Report* 57, no. 45 [November 14, 2008]: 1226–28, www.cdc.gov /mmwr/preview/mmwrhtml/mm5745a3.htm, accessed December 25, 2012).

4. Thomas P. Duffy, "The Flexner Report — 100 Years," *Yale Journal of Biology and Medicine* 84, no. 3 (September 2011): 269–76.

5. E. A. Ferenczi et al., "Can a Statin Neutralize the Cardiovascular Risk of Unhealthy Dietary Choices?," *American Journal of Cardiology* 106, no. 4 (August 15, 2010): 587–92.

6. A. W. Kimball, "Errors of the Third Kind in Statistical Consulting," *Journal of the American Statistical Association* 68, no. 78 (June 1957): 133–42.

7. D. M. Eisenberg et al., "Unconventional Medicine in the United States: Prevalence, Costs, and Patterns of Use," *New England Journal of Medicine* 328, no. 4 (January 28, 1993): 246–52. D. M. Eisenberg et al., "Trends in Alternative Medicine Use in the United States, 1990–1997: Results of a Follow-Up National Survey," *Journal of the American Medical Association* 280, no. 18 (November 11, 1998): 1569–75.

8. "Complementary, Alternative, or Integrative Health: What's in a Name?" October 2008, National Center for Complementary and Alternative Medicine, nccam .nih.gov/health/whatiscam, accessed November 5, 2012.

Chapter 3. A Visit with an Integrative Physician

1. Doctors have big books and checklists to help us come up with a diagnosis. Some of the things on the list are arbitrary. They do change over time, and the diagnostic categories are revised every few years.

2. T. Maus, "Imaging the Back Pain Patient," *Physical Medicine and Rehabilitation Clinics of North America* 21, no. 4 (2010): 725–66. When MRIs are done on normal people with no back pain, a high percentage of them show disc abnormalities that are not causing any symptoms. So what we see on tests is not always the cause of the pain.

3. Quinoa and buckwheat are actually seeds, but people think of them as grain substitutes.

Chapter 4. The Healing Diet

1. W. A. Price, *Nutrition and Physical Degeneration*, 6th ed. (Lemon Grove, CA: Price Pottenger Nutrition Foundation, 2000).

2. In North America, the United States has the worst diet, with Canada faring a little better but following in the United States' footsteps. Mexico has a better, more plant-based diet. However, most of the commercial tortillas available in Mexico are made from genetically modified corn, and the number of US fast-food franchises in Mexico is increasing rapidly.

3. S. Messier et al., "Weight Loss Reduces Knee-Joint Loads in Overweight and Obese Older Adults with Knee Osteoarthritis," *Arthritis and Rheumatism* 52, no. 7 (July 2005): 2026–32.

4. By *farmers*, I mean all food growers. When we think of farms, we tend to think

of the old-fashioned, back-to-the-earth, family operations built and maintained by multigenerational farmers. But in fact much of our food in North America is grown by big corporations, which don't resemble a Norman Rockwell painting in any way. In addition, more than 80 percent of the antibiotics produced by pharmaceutical companies are used in the production of our food. M. Gilchrist et al., "The Potential Role of Concentrated Animal Feeding Operations in Infectious Disease Epidemics and Antibiotic Resistance," *Environmental Health Perspectives* 115, no. 2 (2007): 313–16.

5.   Jennifer L. Harris, Marlene B. Schwartz, and Kelly D. Brownell, *Fast Food Facts: Evaluating Fast Food Nutrition and Marketing to Youth* (New Haven, CT: Yale Rudd Center for Food Policy and Obesity, December 2010), ix, www.fastfood marketing.org/media/FastFoodFACTS_Report.pdf, accessed February 2, 2013. In 1970 Americans spent $6 billion on fast food, and by 2000 they were spending over $110 billion. All indications suggest that the amount has risen since then. E. Schlosser, *Fast Food Nation: The Dark Side of the All-American Meal* (New York: Houghton Mifflin, 2001), 3, http://books.google.com/books?id=yNFN1 OpnkBkC&q=110#v=onepage&q=110&f=false, accessed February 24, 2013.

6.   US Department of Agriculture, "Profiling Food Consumption in America," in *The Agriculture Fact Book, 2001–2002* (Washington, DC: Government Printing Office, 2003), www.usda.gov/factbook/chapter2.pdf, accessed February 14, 2012.

7.   In 2011, the Food Pyramid was replaced with My Plate, which encourages eating more vegetables and suggests that at least half of our grain intake should be whole grains. This means that the USDA still views it as acceptable for half of our grain intake to be composed of high-glycemic, processed grains. The old model still influences nutrition education and advice.

8.   Feed grains, wheat, rice, soybeans, and corn account for the bulk of farm subsidies.

9.   There are other free radicals as well. I use ROS as an example of how all of them function.

10.   N. D. Barnard et al., "A Low-Fat Vegan Diet and a Conventional Diabetes Diet in the Treatment of Type 2 Diabetes: A Randomized, Controlled, 74-Week Clinical Trial," *American Journal of Clinical Nutrition* 89 (2009): 1588S–96S; S. E. Berkow et al., "Diet and Survival after Prostate Cancer Diagnosis," *Nutrition Reviews* 65, no. 9 (2007): 391–403.

11.   Melinda Wenner, "Humans Carry More Bacterial Cells than Human Ones," *Scientific American* (November 30, 2007), www.scientificamerican.com/article .cfm?id=strange-but-true-humans-carry-more-bacterial-cells-than-human-ones, accessed December 28, 2012.

12.   On the Human Microbiome Project, see "Human Microbiome Project," National Institutes of Health, undated, http://commonfund.nih.gov/hmp/, accessed March 1, 2013. On irritable bowel syndrome, see T. S. King, M. Elia, and J. O.

Hunter, "Abnormal Colonic Fermentation in Irritable Bowel Syndrome," *Lancet* 352, no. 9135 (October 10, 1998): 1187–89.

13. The issue of fiber and bowel cancer is controversial; Burkitt associated high fiber with lower cancer rates. Denis Burkitt, *Don't Forget Fibre in Your Diet: To Help Avoid Many of Our Commonest Diseases* (London: Martin Dunitz, 1979).

14. On the association of bowel-movement frequency and cancer, see R. Mody, "P866: Risk of Developing Colorectal Cancer and Benign Neoplasm in Patients with Chronic Constipation" (paper presented at the American College of Gastroenterology Annual Scientific Meeting, October 19–24, 2012, Las Vegas (this was the AGA's annual conference); Dagfinn Aune et al., "Dietary Fibre, Whole Grains, and Risk of Colorectal Cancer: Systematic Review and Dose-Response Meta-analysis of Prospective Studies," *British Medical Journal* 343 (2011): d6617.

15. Technically IBS is a syndrome and not a disease. Studies on GERD and constipation are not yet in the literature. But over the past twenty years, I have found that GERD improves dramatically when constipation is remedied.

16. Stephen A. Hoption Cann, "Hypothesis: Dietary Iodine Intake in the Etiology of Cardiovascular Disease," *Journal of the American College of Nutrition* 25, no. 1 (2006): 1–11.

17. On iodine and breast disease, see S. Venturi, "Is There a Role for Iodine in Breast Diseases?," *Breast* 10, no. 5 (October 2001): 379–82; and S. A. Cann et al., "Hypothesis: Iodine, Selenium and the Development of Breast Cancer," *Cancer Causes Control* 11, no. 2 (February 2000): 121–27. On iodine and ovarian health, see National Institutes of Health, "Iodine," MedlinePlus, undated, www.nlm.nih .gov/medlineplus/druginfo/natural/35.html, accessed March 30, 2013. On iodine and prostate health, see S. A. Hoption Cann, "A Prospective Study of Iodine Status, Thyroid Function, and Prostate Cancer Risk: Follow-Up of the First National Health and Nutrition Examination Survey," *Nutrition and Cancer* 58, no. 1 (2007): 28–34.

18. F. S. Atkinson et al., "International Tables of Glycemic Index and Glycemic Load Values: 2008," *Diabetes Care* 31, no. 12 (December 2008): 2281–83. This article explains the difference between *glycemic index* and *glycemic load* and has an appendix online with lists of the values, which you can look up. See "Supplementary Material: Online-Only Appendix," on p. 3 of www.ncbi.nlm.nih.gov/pmc /articles/PMC2584181/, accessed May 25, 2013.

19. H. Barkoukis et al., "A High Glycemic Meal Suppresses the Postprandial Leptin Response in Normal Healthy Adults," *Annals of Nutrition and Metabolism* 51, no. 6 (December 10, 2007): 512–18.

20. C. Bouché et al., "Five-Week, Low-Glycemic-Index Diet Decreases Total Fat Mass and Improves Plasma Lipid Profile in Moderately Overweight Nondiabetic Men," *Diabetes Care* 25, no. 5 (May 2002): 822–28; A. C. Nilsson, "Effect of

Cereal Test Breakfasts Differing in Glycemic Index and Content of Indigestible Carbohydrates on Daylong Glucose Tolerance in Healthy Subjects," *American Journal of Clinical Nutrition* 87, no. 3 (March 2008): 645–54; Alan W. Barclay et al., "Glycemic Index, Glycemic Load, and Chronic Disease Risk — a Meta-analysis of Observational Studies," *American Journal of Clinical Nutrition* 87, no. 3 (March 2008): 627–37.

21. Frances Moore Lappé, *Diet for a Small Planet* (New York: Ballantine Books, 1991), 121–24.

22. T. C. Campbell and T. M. Campbell, *The China Study: The Most Comprehensive Study of Nutrition Ever Conducted and the Startling Implications for Diet, Weight Loss, and Long-Term Health* (Dallas, TX: BenBella Books, 2005).

23. In 2007 a study was done on the risk of salmonella in eggs produced by chickens in large commercial barns, as compared to the risk in eggs produced by farms raising free-range and organically grown chickens. The risk of salmonella was highest in the large commercial barns. "Report of the Task Force on Zoonoses Data Collection on the Analysis of the Baseline Study on the Prevalence of *Salmonella* in Holdings of Laying Hen Flocks of *Gallus gallus*," *European Food Safety Authority Journal* 97 (2007), www.efsa.europa.eu/en/efsajournal/doc/97r.pdf, accessed June 16, 2013.

24. While Brazil nuts are still healthy, you should not consume more than a few per day, because they contain higher levels of selenium than other nuts do.

25. The best way to prepare nuts is to soak them in water for eight hours to reduce the phytates in them. Phytates can leach minerals from your body and contribute to the development of osteoporosis. The nuts should then be dried at room temperature, in a dehydrator, or in an oven at the lowest temperature, with the door slightly ajar. Dry until the nuts are crispy.

26. I. Staprans et al., "Oxidized Cholesterol in the Diet Accelerates the Development of Atherosclerosis in LDL Receptor- and Apolipoprotein E-Deficient Mice," *Arteriosclerosis, Thrombosis, and Vascular Biology* 20, no. 3 (March 2000): 708–14; G. Spiteller, "The Relation of Lipid Peroxidation Processes with Atherogenesis: A New Theory on Atherogenesis," *Molecular Nutrition and Food Research* 49, no. 11 (November 2005): 999–1013.

27. J. C. Callaway, "Formation of Trans-Fatty Acids in Heated Hempseed Oil: A Rebuttal," www.druglibrary.org/olsen/hemp/iha/jiha5212.html, accessed June 22, 2013. An Li et al., "Thermally Induced Isomerization of Linoleic Acid in Soybean Oil," *Chemistry and Physics of Lipids* 166 (2013): 55–60.

28. Victoria J. Drake, "Nutrition and Inflammation," Linus Pauling Institute, Oregon State University website, last updated August 2010, http://lpi.oregonstate.edu/infocenter/inflammation.html, accessed June 16, 2013.

29. Gamma-linolenic acid is an omega-6 that most people can make from linoleic

acid. A few individuals lack the conversion enzyme and so must get gamma-linolenic acid from food.

30. R. Dufault et al., "Mercury from Chlor-Alkali Plants: Measured Concentrations in Food Product Sugar," *Environmental Health* 8, no. 2 (January 2009).

31. X. Qin, "What Made Canada Become a Country with the Highest Incidence of Inflammatory Bowel Disease: Could Sucralose Be the Culprit?" *Canadian Journal of Gastroenterology* 25, no. 9 (September 2011): 511; M. B. Abou-Donia et al., "Splenda Alters Gut Microflora and Increases Intestinal p-Glycoprotein and Cytochrome p-450 in Male Rats," *Journal of Toxicology and Environmental Health* 71, no. 21 (2008): 1415–29.

32. US Department of Agriculture, "Profiling Food Consumption in America"; New Hampshire Department of Health and Human Services, "How Much Sugar Do You Eat? You May Be Surprised!," DHHS website, 2007, www.dhhs.nh.gov /DPHS/nhp/adults/documents/sugar.pdf, accessed June 16, 2013.

33. C. Colantuoni et al., "Excessive Sugar Intake Alters Binding to Dopamine and Mu-Opioid Receptors in the Brain," *Neuroreport* 12, no. 16 (2001): 3549–52; M. Lenoir et al., "Intense Sweetness Surpasses Cocaine Reward," *PLoS One* 2, no. 8 (2007): e698; A. Gearhardt et al., "Food Addiction, an Examination of the Diagnostic Criteria for Dependence," *Journal of Addiction Medicine* 3 (2009): 1–7.

34. Y. Nakagawa et al., "Sweet Taste Receptor Expressed in Pancreatic b-Cells Activates the Calcium and Cyclic AMP Signaling Systems and Stimulates Insulin Secretion," *PLoS One* 4, no. 4 (2009): 1–11, accessed March 10, 2013.

35. D. Grassi et al., "Blood Pressure Is Reduced and Insulin Sensitivity Increased in Glucose-Intolerant, Hypertensive Subjects after 15 Days of Consuming High-Polyphenol Dark Chocolate," *Journal of Nutrition* 138 (September 2008): 1671–76.

36. Rome Neal, "Caffeine Nation," CBS News, February 11, 2009, www.cbsnews .com/8301-3445_162-529388.html, accessed March 10, 2013.

37. "What Are the Most Commonly Traded Commodities?," InvestorGuide.com, January 25, 2013, www.investorguide.com/igu-article-1139-investing-basics -what-are-the-most-commonly-traded-commodities.html, accessed December 28, 2012.

38. This may be because tea is also an adaptogen, a compound that helps your body deal with stress. This, and the tendency of people to brew tea so it contains less caffeine than the usual cup of coffee, may be what makes it less of a problem for most people.

39. "Benzene Production from Cecarboxylation of Benzoic Acid in the Presence of Ascorbic Acid and a Transition Metal Catalyst," *Journal of Agriculture and Food Chemistry* 141, no. 5 (May 1993): 693–95.

40. Isabel C. Escobar and Andrea Schäfer, *Sustainable Water for the Future: Water*

Recycling versus Desalination, vol. 2, *Sustainability, Science, and Engineering* (Amsterdam: Elsevier, 2010).

41. R. Terry et al., "The Use of Ginger (*Zingiber officinale*) for the Treatment of Pain: A Systematic Review of Clinical Trials," *Pain Medicine* 12, no. 12 (December 2011): 1808–18.

42. Ginger has four different ways to inhibit the enzyme COX 2, which promotes inflammation. R. C. Lantz et al., "The Effect of Extracts from Ginger Rhizome on Inflammatory Mediator Production," *Phytomedicine* 14, no. 2 (February 19, 2007): 123–28.

43. V. Kuptniratsaikul et al., "Efficacy and Safety of *Curcuma domestica* Extracts in Patients with Knee Osteoarthritis," *Journal of Alternative and Complementary Medicine* 15, no. 8 (August 2009): 891–97. When used as an anti-inflammatory, 2,000 mg of turmeric is equal to 800 mg of ibuprofen. K. A. Agarwal et al., "Efficacy of Turmeric (*Curcumin*) in Pain and Postoperative Fatigue after Laparoscopic Cholecystectomy: A Double-Blind, Randomized Placebo-Controlled Study," *Surgical Endoscopy* 25, no. 12 (December 2011): 3805–10.

44. James A. (Jim) Duke, "The Garden Pharmacy: Turmeric, the Queen of COX-2-Inhibitors," *Alternative and Complementary Therapies* 13, no. 5 (October 2007): 229–34.

45. A. M. Roussel et al., "Antioxidant Effects of a Cinnamon Extract in People with Impaired Fasting Glucose That Are Overweight or Obese," *Journal of the American College of Nutrition* 28, no. 1 (February 2009): 16–21; R. Akilen et al., "Glycated Haemoglobin and Blood Pressure–Lowering Effect of Cinnamon in Multi-ethnic Type 2 Diabetic Patients in the UK: A Randomized, Placebo-Controlled, Double-Blind Clinical Trial," *Diabetes Medicine* 27, no. 10 (October 2010): 1159–67, accessed June 16, 2013.

46. Ramón Estruch et al., "Primary Prevention of Cardiovascular Disease with a Mediterranean Diet," *New England Journal of Medicine* 368 (April 4, 2013): 1279–90.

47. G. Schwalfenberg, "The Alkaline Diet: Is There Evidence That an Alkaline pH Diet Benefits Health?," *Journal of Environmental Public Health* (2012), published online in October 2012.

48. S. E. Brown and L. Trivieri Jr., *The Acid-Alkaline Food Guide: A Quick Reference to Foods and Their Effect on pH Levels* (Garden City Park, NY: Square One Publishers, 2006).

49. The part of the gluten that is called gliadin is usually the part people are most sensitive to.

50. A recent study from Spain tested for gluten in oats. It is not totally clear if oats can be eaten by people with celiac disease. A. Real et al., "Molecular and Immunological Characterization of Gluten Proteins Isolated from Oat Cultivars That

Differ in Toxicity for Celiac Disease," *PLoS One* 7, no. 12 (December 2012), www.plosone.org/article/info%3Adoi%2F10.1371%2Fjournal.pone.0048365, accessed July 10, 2013.

51. A. Sapone et al., "Divergence of Gut Permeability and Mucosal Immune Gene Expression in Two Gluten-Associated Conditions: Celiac Disease and Gluten Sensitivity," *BMC Medicine* 9 (March 9, 2011): 23.

Chapter 5. Resolve Stress and Dissolve Pain

1. Descartes's contemporary Galileo was given a life sentence of house arrest for speaking out against church doctrine.

2. Candace Pert and others deliberately mix up the order of the words *mind* and *body* to avoid implying that one is more important than the other.

3. Doc Lew Childre, Howard Martin, and Donna Beech, *The HeartMath Solution: The Institute of HeartMath's Revolutionary Program for Engaging the Power of the Heart's Intelligence* (San Francisco: HarperSanFrancisco, 1999).

4. T. T. MacDonald, "Immunity, Inflammation, and Allergy in the Gut," *Science* 307, no. 5717 (2005): 1920–25.

5. The cortex is the part of the brain that has to do with thought, attention, consciousness, and memory. The limbic system is the part of the brain that affects emotion and long-term memory. The hypothalamic pituitary axis connects the brain to the body through chemical and electrical messages.

6. Hans Selye, *The Stress of Life* (New York: McGraw-Hill, 1984).

7. Hans Selye, MD, researched the stress response with sophisticated studies that looked at healthy and unhealthy stress.

8. J. F. Thayer and E. Sternberg, "Beyond Heart Rate Variability," *Annals of the New York Academy of Sciences* 1088 (November 2006): 361–72.

9. R. Sapolsky, *Why Zebras Don't Get Ulcers: A Guide to Stress, Stress-Related Diseases, and Coping* (New York: Henry Holt, 2004), 101.

10. God "breathed" life into Adam. *Qi*, which means "life force" in Traditional Chinese Medicine, also means breath. *Prana* (from the Vedic tradition of India) refers to both breath and our vital energy.

11. Traditional forms of medicine are holistic and represent "the sum total of knowledge, skills and practices based on the theories, beliefs and experiences indigenous to different cultures that are used to maintain health, as well as to prevent, diagnose, improve or treat physical and mental illnesses," "Traditional Medicine," fact sheet no. 134, World Health Organization, December 2008, www.who.int/mediacentre/factsheets/fs134/en/, accessed May 27, 2013.

12. On reducing anxiety, see P. Carrington et al., "The Use of Meditation-Relaxation Techniques for the Management of Stress in a Working Population," *Journal of Occupational Medicine* 22, no. 4 (April 1980): 222–31. On altering heart function,

see H. Benson, S. Alexander, and C. L. Feldman, "Decreased Premature Ventricular Contractions through the Use of the Relaxation Response in Patients with Stable Ischemic Heart Disease," *Lancet* 2 (1975): 380–82. On lowering blood pressure, see E. Grossman et al., "Breathing-Control Lowers Blood Pressure," *Journal of Human Hypertension* 15, no. 4 (April 2001): 263–69. On reducing the severity of asthma attacks, see S. Cooper et al., "Effect of Two Breathing Exercises (Buteyko and Pranayama) in Asthma: A Randomised Controlled Trial," *Thorax* 58 (2003): 674–79. Further study is needed to confirm the benefits of breathing techniques. On improving the quality of sleep, see G. D. Jacobs, H. Benson, and R. Friedman, "Home-Based Central Nervous System Assessment of Multifactor Behavioral Intervention for Chronic Sleep-Onset Insomnia," *Behavior Therapy* 24 (1993): 159–74.

13. Jon Kabat-Zinn, *Full Catastrophe Living: Using the Wisdom of Your Body and Mind to Face Stress, Pain, and Illness* (New York: Delta, 2005).

14. C. A. Fragoso et al., "Peak Expiratory Flow as a Predictor of Subsequent Disability and Death in Community-Living Older Persons," *Journal of the American Geriatrics Society* 56, no. 6 (June 2008): 1014–20; H. J. Schünemann et al., "Pulmonary Function Is a Long-Term Predictor of Mortality in the General Population: 29-Year Follow-Up of the Buffalo Health Study," *Chest* 118, no. 3 (September 2000): 656–64.

15. Candace Pert, *Molecules of Emotion: The Science behind Mind-Body Medicine* (New York: Simon and Schuster, 1997), 187.

16. This is called entrainment, and it is explained in chapter 6.

17. Kabat-Zinn, *Full Catastrophe Living*.

18. Jon Kabat-Zinn, *Wherever You Go, There You Are* (New York: Hyperion, 1994).

19. R. A. Emmons and M. E. McCullough, "Counting Blessings versus Burdens: Experimental Studies of Gratitude and Subjective Well-Being," *Journal of Personality and Social Psychology* 84 (2003): 377–89.

20. J. Achterberg et al., "Evidence for Correlations between Distant Intentionality and Brain Function in Recipients: A Functional Magnetic Resonance Imaging Analysis," *Journal of Alternative and Complementary Medicine* 11, no. 6 (December 2005): 965–71.

21. M. C. Bushnell, M. Ceko, and L. A. Low, "Cognitive and Emotional Control of Pain and Its Disruption in Chronic Pain," *Nature Reviews Neuroscience* 14, no. 7 (June 2013): 502–11, www.ncbi.nlm.nih.gov/pubmed/?term=bushnell%2C ++meditation, accessed July 12, 2013.

22. L. S. Berk et al., "Neuroendocrine and Stress Hormone Changes during Mirthful Laughter," *American Journal of the Medical Sciences* 298, no. 6 (1989): 390–96.

23. Sven Svebak, Bjorn Kristoffersen, and Knut Aasarod, "Sense of Humor and Survival among a County Cohort of Patients with End-Stage Renal Failure:

A Two-Year Prospective Study," *International Journal of Psychiatry in Medicine* 36, no. 3 (2006): 269–81.

24. Norman Cousins is adjunct professor of Medical Humanities for the School of Medicine at the University of California, Los Angeles, and editor of *Saturday Review*.

25. Alex Cahana, MD, PhD, was the chief of the Division of Pain Medicine at the University of Washington and continues to be a leader in changing the paradigm of pain care.

Chapter 6. Healthy Habits

1. D. S. Ludwig and J. Kabat-Zinn, "Mindfulness in Medicine," *Journal of the American Medical Association* 300, no. 11 (2008): 1350–52; J. Kabat-Zinn and R. Burney, "The Clinical Use of Awareness Meditation in the Self-Regulation of Chronic Pain," *Pain* 11, suppl. 1 (1981): S273.

2. R. Doll et al., "Mortality in Relation to Smoking: 50 Years' Observations on Male British Doctors," *British Medical Journal* 328 (June 2004): 1519.

3. Malcolm Gladwell, *The Tipping Point: How Little Things Can Make a Big Difference* (Little, Brown, 2002), 216–52.

4. "2012 Bedroom Poll," National Sleep Foundation, www.sleepfoundation.org /sites/default/files/bedroom2012.pdf, accessed June 16, 2013.

5. "Women and Sleep," National Sleep Foundation, undated, www.sleepfoundation .org/article/sleep-topics/women-and-sleep, accessed June 16, 2013; "Insomnia," Mayo Clinic, January 2, 2011, www.mayoclinic.com/health/insomnia/DS00187 /DSECTION=causes, accessed June 16, 2013.

6. "The zone" is described by athletes and experienced by many people as a state in which they feel their mental and physical state is optimally focused for the task at hand. M. Lardon, *Finding Your Zone* (New York: Penguin, 2008).

7. Doc Lew Childre, Howard Martin, and Donna Beech, *The HeartMath Solution: The Institute of HeartMath's Revolutionary Program for Engaging the Power of the Heart's Intelligence* (San Francisco: HarperSanFrancisco, 1999).

8. D. E. Blask et al., "Putting Cancer to Sleep at Night," *Endocrine* 27, no. 2 (July 2005): 179–88; A. Carillo-Vico et al., "A Review of the Multiple Actions of Melatonin on the Immune System," *Endocrine* 27, no. 2 (July 2005): 189–200; C. Cirelli and G. Tononi, "Is Sleep Essential?," *PLoS Biology* 6, no. 8 (August 2008), www.plosbiology.org/article/info:doi/10.1371/journal.pbio.0060216, accessed May 27, 2013.

9. A. Pack, "The Gears of the Sleep Clock," *Scientist* (April 1, 2009), www.the -scientist.com/?articles.view/articleNo/27239/title/The-Gears-of-the-Sleep -Clock/, accessed May 27, 2013.

10. A. R. Ekirch, *At Day's Close: Night in Times Past* (New York: Norton, 2005).

11. T. A. Wehr, "In Short Photoperiods, Human Sleep Is Biphasic," *Journal of Sleep Research* 1, no. 2 (June 1992): 103–7.

12. Rubin R. Naiman, *Healing Night: The Science and Spirit of Sleeping, Dreaming, and Awakening* (Minneapolis, MN: Syren Book Company, 2006).

13. Norwegian Ministry of the Environment, "Dental Mercury Use Banned in Norway, Sweden and Denmark Because Composites Are Adequate," press release, January 3, 2008, Reuters, www.reuters.com/article/2008/01/03/idUS108558+03-Jan-2008+PRN20080103, accessed May 27, 2013.

14. "Mercury in Health Care," World Health Organization, 2005, www.who.int/water_sanitation_health/medicalwaste/mercurypolpap230506.pdf, accessed July 10, 2013. Two more recent documents speak about phasing out mercury: "WHO Welcomes International Treaty on Mercury," World Health Organization, January 19, 2013, www.who.int/mediacentre/news/statements/2013/mercury_20130119/en; and United Nations Environment Programme, *Mercury: Time to Act* (Geneva: UNEP, 2013), www.unep.org/PDF/PressReleases/Mercury_TimeToAct.pdf, both accessed May 27, 2013.

15. Janet Travell, MD, described this phenomenon during a course on myofascial pain that I attended in the early 1990s.

16. "Tend and Befriend," UCLA Social Neuroscience Lab, undated, http://taylorlab.psych.ucla.edu/research.htm, accessed June 1, 2013.

17. Brian Sutton-Smith, *The Ambiguity of Play* (Cambridge, MA: Harvard University Press, 2001).

18. Deepak Chopra, "Gratitude Is the Highest Point of View," *Chopra Center Newsletter*, November 2011, www.chopra.com/files/newsletter/Nov11/Newsletter-Nov11-deepak.html, accessed April 25, 2013.

19. Our nature is what we were born with as a temperament, and nurture is what we have learned through experiences in our lives.

20. For information about this field of psychology, see the Authentic Happiness website, www.authentichappiness.sas.upenn.edu.

21. The happiest people lived into their nineties. Daniel Tomasulo, "Proof Positive: Can Heaven Help Us? The Nun Study — Afterlife," Psych Central, undated, http://psychcentral.com/blog/archives/2010/10/27/proof-positive-can-heaven-help-us-the-nun-study-afterlife/, accessed May 27, 2013.

22. E. S. Ford et al., "Healthy Living Is the Best Revenge: Findings from the European Prospective Investigation into Cancer and Nutrition — Potsdam Study," *Archives of Internal Medicine* 169, no. 15 (2009): 1355–62.

Chapter 7. Dietary Supplements

1. A. C. Bronstein et al., "2010 Annual Report of the American Association of Poison Control Centers' National Poison Data System (NPDS): 28th Annual

Report," *Clinical Toxicology* (Philadelphia) 49, no. 10 (2011): 910–41, www.ncbi
.nlm.nih.gov/pubmed/22165864, accessed June 16, 2013.

Based on this report there were no deaths due to multiple vitamins, A, B, C, D, E, or any other vitamin, and no deaths attributable to amino acid or other dietary supplements. Very often allopathic medicine treats recommendations to take vitamins with more caution than recommendations to take drugs or have surgery. I showed in chapter 2 that our allopathic health care system causes hundreds of thousands of deaths each year. Here I am purposely reporting the number of deaths from taking vitamins (zero) as a direct comparison for my critics.

2. R. Williams, *Biochemical Individuality*, 2nd ed. (New York: McGraw-Hill, 1998).

3. As defined in the Institute of Medicine, *Dietary Reference Intakes: A Risk Assessment Model for Establishing Upper Intake Levels for Nutrients* (Washington, DC: National Academies Press, 1998), 3, www.nap.edu/openbook.php?record_id=6432&page=3, accessed June 21, 2013.

4. R. Löbenberg and W. Steinke, "Investigation of Vitamin and Mineral Tablets and Capsules on the Canadian Market," *Journal of Pharmacy and Pharmaceutical Sciences* 9, no. 1 (2006): 40–49.

5. Both Good Manufacturing Practices and International Organization for Standardization offer guidelines for production and testing to help to ensure a quality product.

6. NSF.com and Consumerlab.com are two websites that test products and list the results on their websites, to which you can subscribe.

7. R. D. Donald, "Changes in USDA Food Composition Data for 43 Garden Crops, 1950 to 1999," *Journal of the American College of Nutrition* 23, no. 6 (2004): 669–82.

8. S. Boyd Eaton, "The Ancestral Human Diet: What Was It and Should It Be a Paradigm for Contemporary Nutrition?" *Proceedings of the Nutrition Society* 65, no. 1 (February 2006): 1–6.

9. A excellent explanation of the growing problem of malnutrition in the midst of plenty in the United States can be seen in the film *A Place at the Table*, directed by Kristi Jacobson and Lori Silverbush, www.magpictures.com/aplaceatthetable/.

10. F. Vagnini and B. Fox, *The Side Effects Bible* (New York: Broadway Books, 2005); R. Pelton et al., Drug-Induced Nutrient Depletion Handbook, 1999–2000 (Hudson, OH: Lexi-Comp, 1999).

11. Qun Xu et al., "Multivitamin Use and Telomere Length in Women," *American Journal of Clinical Nutrition* 89, no. 6 (June 2009): 1857–63.

12. Bruce N. Ames, "A Role for Supplements in Optimizing Health: The Metabolic Tune-Up," *Archives of Biochemistry and Biophysics* 423, no. 1 (March 1, 2004): 227–34.

13. Satomi Ohsako and Keith B. Elkon, "Apoptosis in the Effector Phase of Autoimmune Diabetes, Multiple Sclerosis and Thyroiditis," *Cell Death and Differentiation* 6, no. 1 (1998): 13.

14.   S. Maggini et al., "Selected Vitamins and Trace Elements Support Immune Function by Strengthening Epithelial Barriers and Cellular and Humoral Immune Responses," *British Journal of Nutrition* 98, suppl. 1 (October 2007): S29–S35.

15.   K. M. Fairfield and R. H. Fletcher, "Vitamins for Chronic Disease Prevention in Adults: Scientific Review," *Journal of the American Medical Association* 287, no. 23 (June 19, 2002): 3116–26, 3127–29.

16.   M. Shargorodsky et al., "Effect of Long-Term Treatment with Antioxidants (Vitamin C, Vitamin E, Coenzyme Q_{10} and Selenium) on Arterial Compliance, Humoral Factors and Inflammatory Markers in Patients with Multiple Cardiovascular Risk Factors," *Nutrition and Metabolism* (London) 7 (July 6, 2010): 55.

17.   High doses of supplements of beta-carotene have been shown to have negative effects on smokers with lung cancer. This does not hold true for food sources of beta-carotene.

18.   It is especially important to limit the amount of retinol taken during pregnancy to its RDA.

19.   Restless leg syndrome is characterized by the need to move your legs to relieve unpleasant sensations. It typically occurs at night.

20.   K. S. McCully, *The Homocysteine Revolution Medicine for the New Millennium* (Lincolnwood, IL: Keats, 1999).

21.   L. Wyatt et al., "Efficacy of Vitamin B-6 in the Treatment of Premenstrual Syndrome: Systematic Review," *British Medical Journal* 318, no. 7195 (May 22, 1999): 1375–81.

22.   J. Schoenen, J. Jacquy, and M. Lenaerts, "Effectiveness of High-Dose Riboflavin in Migraine Prophylaxis: A Randomized Controlled Trial," *Neurology* 50, no. 2 (1998): 466–70.

23.   G. L. Mauro et al., "Vitamin B12 in Low Back Pain: A Randomised, Double-Blind, Placebo-Controlled Study," *European Review for Medical and Pharmacological Sciences* 4, no. 3 (May–June 2000): 53–58.

24.   Jane Higdon, "Vitamin C," Linus Pauling Institute, Oregon State University website, last updated November 2009, http://lpi.oregonstate.edu/infocenter/vitamins/vitaminC/.

25.   R. J. Jariwalla and S. Harakeh, "Antiviral and Immunomodulatory Activities of Ascorbic Acid," in *Subcellular Biochemistry*, vol. 25, *Ascorbic Acid: Biochemistry and Biomedical Cell Biology*, ed. J. R. Harris (New York: Plenum Press, 1996), 215–31.

26.   J. A. Simon and E. S. Hudes, "Relationship of Ascorbic Acid to Blood Lead Levels," *Journal of the American Medical Association* 281, no. 24 (1999): 2289–93.

27.   Vitamin D is actually best regarded as a hormone, an internal communication molecule.

28. D. D. Bikle, "Vitamin D and Immune Function: Understanding Common Pathways," *Current Osteoporosis Reports* 7, no. 2 (July 2009): 58–63.
29. T. Takiishi et al., "Vitamin D and Diabetes," *Endocrinology and Metabolism Clinics of North America* 39, no. 2 (June 2010): 419–46.
30. A. S. Grimaldi et al., "25(OH) Vitamin D Is Associated with Greater Muscle Strength in Healthy Men and Women," *Medicine and Science in Sports and Exercise* 45, no. 1 (January 2013): 157–62.
31. M. F. Holick, "Vitamin D Deficiency," *New England Journal of Medicine* 357, no. 3 (July 19, 2007): 266–81; M. Z. Erkal et al., "High Prevalence of Vitamin D Deficiency, Secondary Hyperparathyroidism and Generalized Bone Pain in Turkish Immigrants in Germany: Identification of Risk Factors," *Osteoporosis International* 17, no. 8 (2006): 1133–40; M. K. Turner et al., "Prevalence and Clinical Correlates of Vitamin D Inadequacy among Patients with Chronic Pain," *Pain Medicine* 9, no. 8 (November 2008): 979–84.
32. Holick, "Vitamin D Deficiency."
33. A. C. Helmer and C. H. Jensen, "Vitamin D Precursors Removed from the Skin by Washing," *Studies Institute Divi Thomae* 1 (1937): 207–16, as discussed on the Vitamin D Council website, www.vitamindcouncil.org.
34. The table is based on information supplied by the Vitamin D Council website, "Testing for Vitamin D," www.vitamindcouncil.org/about-vitamin-d/testing-for-vitamin-d, accessed June 30, 2013.
35. J. J. Cannell, "Vitamin D and the Chicago Blackhawks," *Vitamin D Council Newsletter*, May 2010, www.vitamindcouncil.org/?o=1395, accessed April 6, 2013.
36. S. Lemaire-Ewing et al., "Vitamin E Transport, Membrane Incorporation and Cell Metabolism: Is Alpha-Tocopherol in Lipid Rafts an Oar in the Lifeboat?," *Molecular Nutrition and Food Research* 54, no. 5 (May 2010): 631–40.
37. M. J. Bolland et al., "Effect of Calcium Supplements on Risk of Myocardial Infarction and Cardiovascular Events: Meta-analysis," *British Medical Journal* 341 (July 29, 2010): c3691.
38. Jane Higdon, "Magnesium," Linus Pauling Institute, Oregon State University website, last updated August 2007, http://lpi.oregonstate.edu/infocenter/minerals/magnesium/, accessed March 30, 2013.
39. D. J. Kim et al., "Magnesium Intake in Relation to Systemic Inflammation, Insulin Resistance, and the Incidence of Diabetes," *Diabetes Care* 33, no. 12 (December 2010): 2604–10.
40. M. Seelig, "Cardiovascular Consequences of Magnesium Deficiency and Loss: Pathogenesis, Prevalence and Manifestations — Magnesium and Chloride Loss in Refractory Potassium Repletion," *American Journal of Cardiology* 63, no. 14 (April 18, 1989): 4G–21G; S. Demirkaya et al., "Efficacy of Intravenous Magnesium Sulfate in the Treatment of Acute Migraine Attacks," *Headache* 41, no. 2

(2001): 171–77; Alexander Mauskop and Jasmine Varughese, "Why All Migraine Patients Should Be Treated with Magnesium," *Journal of Neural Transmission* 119, no. 5 (2012): 575–79.

41. K. Murakami et al., "Association between Dietary Fiber, Water and Magnesium Intake and Functional Constipation among Young Japanese Women," *European Journal of Clinical Nutrition* 61, no. 5 (2007): 616–22.

42. F. H. Nielsen, L. K. Johnson, and H. Zeng, "Magnesium Supplementation Improves Indicators of Low Magnesium Status and Inflammatory Stress in Adults Older Than 51 Years with Poor Quality Sleep," *Magnesium Research* 23, no. 4 (2010): 158–68; L. J. Rondón et al., "Magnesium Attenuates Chronic Hypersensitivity and Spinal Cord NMDA Receptor Phosphorylation in a Rat Model of Diabetic Neuropathic Pain," *Journal of Physiology* 588 (2010): 4205–15; S. Brill et al., "Efficacy of Intravenous Magnesium in Neuropathic Pain," *British Journal of Anaesthesia* 89, no. 5 (2002): 711–14.

43. R. Whang, "Magnesium Deficiency: Pathogenesis, Prevalence, and Clinical Implications," *American Journal of Medicine* 82, no. 3A (March 20, 1987): 24–29.

44. Other forms may stay in the bowels and not help out your muscles.

45. E. L. Prien Sr. and S. N. Gershoff, "Magnesium Oxide-Pyridoxine Therapy for Recurrent Calcium Oxalate Calculi," *Journal of Urology* 112, no. 4 (1974): 509–12.

46. R. Nahas and M. Moher, "Complementary and Alternative Medicine for the Treatment of Type 2 Diabetes," *Canadian Family Physician (Le Médecin de Famille Canadien)* 55, no. 6 (2009): 591–96.

47. Jane Higdon, "Iodine," Linus Pauling Institute, Oregon State University website, last updated March 2010, lpi.oregonstate.edu/infocenter/minerals/iodine/index .html#rda, accessed January 27, 2013.

48. It has been noted in the past that there is an increase of breast disease, including cancer, in women with hypothyroidism. Some research from the 1960s is now being looked at again to show a connection.

49. Iron-containing supplements are also a common cause of household poisonings of children.

50. Y. H. Lee et al., "Omega-3 Polyunsaturated Fatty Acids and the Treatment of Rheumatoid Arthritis: A Meta-analysis," *Archives of Medical Research* 43, no. 5 (July 2012): 356–62; R. J. Goldberg and J. Katz, "A Meta-analysis of the Analgesic Effects of Omega-3 Polyunsaturated Fatty Acid Supplementation for Inflammatory Joint Pain," *Pain* 129 (2007): 210–23.

51. Take the number of milligrams of the entire fish oil pill and divide by the total milligrams of the DHA plus EPA. If the answer is around 2 or less, it is a good-quality fish oil.

52. A. P. Simopoulos, A. Leaf, and N. Salem Jr., "Workshop Statement on the Essentiality of and Recommended Dietary Intakes for Omega-6 and Omega-3 Fatty

Acids," *Prostaglandins, Leukotrienes and Essential Fatty Acids* 63, no. 3 (2000): 119–21; P. M. Kris-Etherton, W. S. Harris, and L. J. Appel, "Fish Consumption, Fish Oil, Omega-3 Fatty Acids, and Cardiovascular Disease," *Circulation* 106, no. 21 (2002): 2747–57.

53. "S-Adenosyl-L-Methionine (SAMe): An Introduction," National Center for Complementary and Alternative Medicine, October 2012, http://nccam.nih.gov /health/supplements/SAMe, accessed May 2013.

54. R. Agosti et al., "Effectiveness of *Petasites hybridus* in the Prophlyaxis of Migraine: A Systematic Review," *Phytomedicine* 13, no. 9–10 (2006): 743–46; A. Schapowal, "Randomized Controlled Trial of Butterbur and Cetitizine for Treating Seasonal Allergic Rhinitis," *British Medical Journal* 324, no. 7330 (2002): 144–46.

55. C. de Filippo et al., "Impact of Diet in Shaping Gut Microbiota Revealed by a Comparative Study in Children from Europe and Rural Africa," *Proceedings of the National Academy of Sciences of the United States of America* 107, no. 33 (2010): 14691–96.

56. US Department of Agriculture and US Department of Health and Human Services, *Dietary Guidelines for Americans 2010*, 7th ed. (Washington, DC: US Government Printing Office, December 2010), www.health.gov/dietaryguide lines/dga2010/DietaryGuidelines2010.pdf, accessed May 15, 2013; Y. Park et al., "Dietary Fiber Intake and Risk of Colorectal Cancer: A Pooled Analysis of Prospective Cohort Studies," *Journal of the American Medical Association* 294, no. 22 (2005): 2849–57.

57. G. Klein et al., "Efficacy and Tolerance of an Oral Enzyme Combination in Painful Osteoarthritis of the Hip: A Double-Blind, Randomised Study Comparing Oral Enzymes with Non-steroidal Anti-inflammatory Drugs. *Clinical and Experimental Rheumatology* 24, no. 1 (January–February 2006): 25–30.

58. M. Loes and D. Steinman, *The Aspirin Alternative: The Natural Way to Overcome Chronic Pain, Reduce Inflammation and Enhance the Healing Response* (Topanga, CA: Freedom Press, 2001).

59. S. Brien et al., "Bromelain as an Adjunctive Treatment for Moderate-to-Severe Osteoarthritis of the Knee: A Randomized Placebo-Controlled Pilot Study," *Quarterly Journal of Medicine* 99, no. 12 (December 2006): 841–50.

60. J. V. Wright, *Dr. Wright's Guide to Healing with Nutrition* (New Canaan, CT: Keats, 1990), 155.

61. H. G. Grigoleit and P. Grigoleit, "Peppermint Oil in Irritable Bowel Syndrome," *Phytomedicine* 12, no. 8 (August 2005): 601–6.

62. K. L. Wu et al., "Effects of Ginger on Gastric Emptying and Motility in Healthy Humans," *European Journal of Gastroenterology and Hepatology* 20, no. 5 (May 2008): 436–40.

63. R. D. Altman, "Effects of a Ginger Extract on Knee Pain in Patients with Osteo-arthritis," *Arthritis and Rheumatism* 44, no. 11 (November 1, 2001): 2531–38.

64. Jody Noé, "L-Glutamine Use in the Treatment and Prevention of Mucositis and Cachexia: A Naturopathic Perspective," *Integrative Cancer Therapies* 8, no. 4 (2009): 409–15.

65. L. Vahdat et al., "Reduction of Paclitaxel-Induced Peripheral Neuropathy with Glutamine," *Clinical Cancer Research* 7, no. 5 (2001): 1192–97.

66. J. Wang et al., "Gene Expression Is Altered in Piglet Small Intestine by Weaning and Dietary Glutamine Supplementation," *Journal of Nutrition* 138, no. 6 (2008): 1025–32.

67. M. Comalada et al., "In Vivo Quercitrin Anti-inflammatory Effect Involves Release of Quercetin, Which Inhibits Inflammation through Down-Regulation of the NF-kappaB Pathway," *European Journal of Immunology* 35, no. 2 (2005): 584–92; Agnes W. Boots et al., "Health Effects of Quercetin: From Antioxidant to Nutraceutical," *European Journal of Pharmacology* 585, no. 2–3 (2008); Daniel A. Valério et al., "Quercetin Reduces Inflammatory Pain: Inhibition of Oxidative Stress and Cytokine Production," *Journal of Natural Products* 72, no. 11 (2009): 1975–79.

68. T. A. Pham-Marcou et al., "Antinociceptive Effect of Resveratrol in Carrageenan-Evoked Hyperagesia in Rats: Prolonged Effect Related to COX-2 Expression Impairment," *Pain* 140, no. 2 (November 30, 2008): 274–83; S. C. Woo et al., "Resveratrol Inhibits Nicotinic Stimulation-Evoked Catecholamine Release from the Adrenal Medulla," *Korean Journal of Physiology and Pharmacology* 12, no. 4 (August 2008): 155–64.

69. "WHO Monographs on Selected Medicinal Plants," vol. 2, World Health Organization, 2004, http://apps.who.int/medicinedocs/en/d/Js4927e/29.html #Js4927e.29, accessed April 21, 2013.

70. There are two forms of alpha-lipoic acid, and they are mirror images of each other. They are called R and L forms. When combined, they are called a racemic mixture. Most studies done on alpha-lipoic acid are done on racemic mixtures. Nevertheless, the R form may be more efficient, while the L form is considered inactive. When choosing alpha-lipoic supplements, look for one with more of the R form.

Chapter 8. Exercise

1. It may actually be a combination of muscle memory and nervous system memory. This may be another example of neuroplasticity.

2. I. P. Rolf, *Rolfing: Reestablishing the Natural Alignment and Structural Integration of the Human Body for Vitality and Well-Being* (Rochester, VT: Healing Arts Press, 1989); J. Travell and D. Simons, *Myofascial Pain and Dysfunction: The*

Trigger Point Manual, 2 vols. (Baltimore: Williams and Wilkins, 1992); T. Myers, *Anatomy Trains: Myofascial Meridians for Manual and Movement Therapists* (Philadelphia: Churchill Livingstone, 2001).

3. S. McGill, *Low Back Disorders, Evidence Based Prevention and Rehabilitation* (Champaign, IL: Human Kinetics, 2002).

4. "Yoga for Health," National Center for Complementary and Alternative Medicine, last updated May 2012, http://nccam.nih.gov/health/yoga/introduction.htm, accessed November 12, 2012.

5. "Tai Chi and Qi Gong for Health and Well-Being," video, National Center for Complementary and Alternative Medicine, undated, http://nccam.nih.gov/video/taichiDVD, accessed November 12, 2012.

Chapter 9. Prescription Drugs

1. Some drugs are lifesaving and should not be stopped without consulting your physician. These include some heart medications, blood pressure medications, and others. Insulin corrects a deficiency and is lifesaving.

2. Peter Jüni et al., "Risk of Cardiovascular Events and Rofecoxib: Cumulative Meta-analysis," *Lancet* 364, no. 9450 (December 4, 2004): 2021–29.

3. Consumers Union, "Testimony of David J. Graham, MD, MPH (November 18, 2004)," www.consumersunion.org/pub/core_health_care/001651.html, accessed April 2, 2013. Graham is associate director for science and medicine in the FDA's Office of Drug Safety, and he testified before the US Senate Committee on Finance.

4. Eric J. Topol, "Failing the Public Health — Rofecoxib, Merck, and the FDA," *New England Journal of Medicine* 351, no. 17 (October 21, 2004).

5. Revenue figures have been dropping since 2008 because of lower-cost generics and not because of fewer prescriptions. Matthew Herper, "Statins Dethroned," Forbes.com, March 30, 2009, www.forbes.com/2009/03/30/statins-heart-disease-business-healthcare-statins.html, accessed March 10, 2013.

6. Acute tendinitis can be helped with anti-inflammatories in the first few weeks if the tendon is red, hot, and swollen. In the later stages anti-inflammatories are not helpful and may actually delay healing.

7. T. J. Kaptchuk et al., "Placebos without Deception: A Randomized Controlled Trial in Irritable Bowel Syndrome," *PLoS One* 5, no. 12 (2010): 1–7.

8. Ernest Lawrence Rossi, *The Psychobiology of Mind-Body Healing: New Concepts of Therapeutic Hypnosis* (New York: Norton, 1993), 18.

9. Aspirin is still safe to take after a heart attack.

10. Anne-Marie Schjerning Olsen et al., "Long-Term Cardiovascular Risk of Nonsteroidal Anti-inflammatory Drug Use According to Time Passed after

First-Time Myocardial Infarction: A Nationwide Cohort Study," *Circulation* 126, no. 16 (October 16, 2012): 1955–63

11. J. P. O'Connor and T. Lysz, "Celecoxib, NSAIDs and the Skeleton," *Drugs of Today* (Barcelona) 44, no. 9 (September 2008): 693–709.

12. G. Obeid, X. Zhang, and X. Wang, "Effect of Ibuprofen on the Healing and Remodeling of Bone and Articular Cartilage in the Rabbit Temporomandibular Joint," *Journal of Oral and Maxillofacial Surgery* 50, no. 8 (1992): 843–49.

13. There are different types of steroids, including anabolic steroids and others.

14. Crystals precipitate out of the solution of the steroid and become irritating to the tissues they are in.

15. Adrenal depletion or fatigue happens because of excess stress and chronic illnesses. Fibromyalgia is usually accompanied by adrenal fatigue.

16. International Narcotics Control Board and United Nations, *Narcotic Drugs Estimated World Requirements for 2011, Statistics for 2009* (New York: United Nations, 2011), http://search.ebscohost.com/login.aspx?direct=true&scope=site&db=nlebk&db=nlabk&AN=387612; Centers for Disease Control and Prevention, National Center for Injury Prevention and Control, *Policy Impact: Prescription Painkiller Overdoses*, CDC website, November 2011, www.cdc.gov /HomeandRecreationalSafety/pdf/PolicyImpact-PrescriptionPainKillerOD .pdf, accessed March 30, 2013; Centers for Disease Control and Prevention, "CDC Grand Rounds: Prescription Drug Overdoses — a U.S. Epidemic," *Morbidity and Mortality Weekly Report* 61, no. 1 (January 13, 2012): 10–13, www.cdc.gov /mmwr/preview/mmwrhtml/mm6101a3.htm, accessed March 31, 2013; Centers for Disease Control and Prevention, National Center for Injury Prevention and Control, "Unintentional Drug Poisoning in the United States," July 2010, www.cdc.gov/HomeandRecreationalSafety/pdf/poison-issue-brief.pdf, accessed March 31, 2013.

17. According to researcher Mary Jeanne Kreek and her colleagues, "Family and twin epidemiological studies show that genes contribute to the vulnerability to addictive disease, with estimates of heritability of 30–60%." "Genetic Influences on Impulsivity, Risk Taking, Stress Responsivity and Vulnerability to Drug Abuse and Addiction," *Nature Neuroscience* 8, no. 11 (November 2005): 1450.

18. J. C. Fournier et al., "Antidepressant Drug Effects and Depression Severity: A Patient-Level Meta-analysis," *Journal of the American Medical Association* 303, no. 1 (2010): 47–53, jama.jamanetwork.com/article.aspx?articleid=185157, accessed March 31, 2013; I. Kirsch et al., "Initial Severity and Antidepressant Benefits: A Meta-analysis of Data Submitted to the Food and Drug Administration," *PLoS Medicine* 5, no. 2 (2008): 260–68, www.plosmedicine.org/article/info:doi /10.1371/journal.pmed.0050045, accessed March 31, 2013; J. H. Meyer et al.,

"Brain Monoamine Oxidase: A Binding in Major Depressive Disorder," *Archives of General Psychiatry* 66, no. 12 (2009): 1304–12.

19. I. Kirsch, *The Emperor's New Drugs: Exploding the Antidepressant Myth* (New York: Random House, 2010).

20. M. Priya et al., "Screening of Cetirizine for Analgesic Activity in Mice," *International Journal of Basic and Clinical Pharmacology* 2, no. 2 (2013): 188.

21. Not every case of repetitive strain injury needs these drugs. I use them if the other treatments, like massage and Gunn IMS, are not working well enough, and if the patient's hands get particularly cold and painful with stress or exposure to cold temperatures. See chapter 11 for more information on treatments.

22. Restless leg syndrome is characterized by the need to move your legs to relieve unpleasant sensations. It typically occurs at night.

23. R. W. Loftus et al., "Intraoperative Ketamine Reduces Perioperative Opiate Consumption in Opiate-Dependent Patients with Chronic Back Pain Undergoing Back Surgery," *Anesthesiology* 113, no. 3 (2010): 639–46; R. F. Kwok et al., "Preoperative Ketamine Improves Postoperative Analgesia after Gynecologic Laparoscopic Surgery," *Anesthesia and Analgesia* 98, no. 4 (2004): 1044–49; Mary Elizabeth Lynch et al., "Topical Amitriptyline and Ketamine in Neuropathic Pain Syndromes: An Open-Label Study," *Journal of Pain* 6, no. 10 (2005): 644–49.

24. This is done at "compounding pharmacies."

25. S. Y. Yoon et al., " An Increase in Spinal Dehydroepiandrosterone Sulfate (DHEAS) Enhances NMDA-Induced Pain via Phosphorylation of the NR1 Subunit in Mice: Involvement of the Sigma-1 Receptor," *Neuropharmacology* 59, no. 6 (November 2010): 460–67.

26. K. G. Sorwell and H. F. Urbanski, "Dehydroepiandrosterone and Age-Related Cognitive Decline," *Age* (Dordrecht) 32, no. 1 (March 2010): 61–67; J. K. van Niekerk, F. A. Huppert, and J. Herbert, "Salivary Cortisol and DHEA: Association with Measures of Cognition and Well-Being in Normal Older Men, and Effects of Three Months of DHEA Supplementation," *Psychoneuroendocrinology* 26, no. 6 (2001): 591–612.

27. A. M. Aloisi et al., "Chronic Pain Therapy and Hypothalamic-Pituitary-Adrenal Axis Impairment," *Psychoneuroendocrinology* 36, no. 7 (2011): 1032–39; J. D. Kilts et al., "Neurosteroids and Self-Reported Pain in Veterans Who Served in the U.S. Military after September 11, 2001," *Pain Medicine* (Malden, MA) 11, no. 10 (2010): 1469–76.

28. W. Mayo et al., "Pregnenolone Sulfate Enhances Neurogenesis and PSA-NCAM in Young and Aged Hippocampus," *Neurobiology of Aging* 26, no. 1 (2005): 103–14.

29. R. Sapolsky, *Why Zebras Don't Get Ulcers: A Guide to Stress, Stress-Related Diseases, and Coping* (New York: Holt, 2004), 296.

258   HOLISTIC PAIN RELIEF

30. DHEA can predict how patients will do in the long run. H. M. Hasselhorn, T. Theorell, and E. Vingård, "Endocrine and Immunologic Parameters Indicative of 6-Month Prognosis after the Onset of Low Back Pain or Neck/Shoulder Pain," *Spine* 26, no. 3 (2001): 24–29; E. Gąsińska et al., "Influence of Acute and Subchronic Oral Administration of Dehydroepiandrosterone (DHEA) on Nociceptive Threshold in Rats," *Pharmacological Reports* 64, no. 4 (2012): 965–69; Yoon, "An Increase in Spinal Dehydroepiandrosterone Sulfate (DHEAS) Enhances NMDA-Induced Pain via Phosphorylation of the NR1 Subunit in Mice."

31. M. E. Dawson-Basoa and A. R. Gintzler, "Estrogen and Progesterone Activate Spinal Kappa-Opiate Receptor Analgesic Mechanisms," *Pain* 64, no. 1 (January 1996): 608–15.

32. C. A. Frye and A. A. Walf, "Estrogen and/or Progesterone Administered Systemically or to the Amygdala Can Have Anxiety-, Fear-, and Pain-Reducing Effects in Ovariectomized Rats," *Behavioral Neuroscience* 118, no. 2 (2004): 306–13.

33. Perimenopause is the time around menopause when symptoms of hormone change begin. This may start ten years before actual cessation of periods marks the start of menopause.

34. J. C. Prior and C. L. Hitchcock, "The Endocrinology of Perimenopause: Need for a Paradigm Shift," *Frontiers in Bioscience* (Scholar edition) 1, no. 3 (January 2011): 474–86.

35. The standard medical protocol is to use progesterone only if the woman still has a uterus, because estrogen alone can cause cancer of the uterus. Once she had a hysterectomy, doctors thought, progesterone would not be necessary. Partly they concluded this because they were using a (synthetic) progestin, which is a nasty drug and not natural progesterone. They were also not aware of the need to balance estrogen with natural progesterone levels. John Lee, *What Your Doctor May Not Tell You about Menopause* (New York: Warner, 2004); J. Wright and J. Morgenthaler, *Natural Hormone Replacement for Women over 45* (Petaluma, CA: Smart Publications, 1997).

36. V. Seifert-Klauss et al., "Progesterone and Bone: A Closer Link Than Previously Realized," *Climacteric* 15, no. S1 (2012): S26–S31; Anne Caufriez et al., "Progesterone Prevents Sleep Disturbances and Modulates GH, TSH and Melatonin Secretion in Postmenopausal Women," *Journal of Clinical Endocrinology and Metabolism* 96, no. 4 (2011): 614–23, http://hdl.handle.net/2013/ULB-DIPOT:oai:dipot.ulb.ac.be:2013/95407.

37. E. Leonelli et al., "Progesterone and Its Derivatives Are Neuroprotective Agents in Experimental Diabetic Neuropathy: A Multimodal Analysis," *Neuroscience* 144, no. 4 (2007): 1293–304; M. Schumacher et al., "Local Synthesis and Dual Actions

of Progesterone in the Nervous System: Neuroprotection and Myelination," *Growth Hormone and IGF Research* 14, suppl. A (June 2004): S18–S33.

38. It is likely also the case that there are microscopic nests of cancer cells in the breasts of most women past a certain age. The immune system keeps these cells in check. We do not yet have ways of figuring out which nests of prostate or breast cancer cells will become a threat to life and which will just stay quiet for the lifetime of the host. P. C. Gøtzsche and M. Nielsen, "Screening for Breast Cancer with Mammography," *Cochrane Database of Systematic Reviews*, no. 4 (October 18, 2006): CD001877; update in *Cochrane Database of Systematic Reviews*, no. 1 (January 19, 2011): CD001877.

39. There is an organization devoted to antiaging medicine that advocates the use of growth-hormone injections. Most integrative physicians use the term *healthy aging* and prefer to increase the patient's own growth-hormone production.

40. When you are stressed for a long time, the morning peak of cortisol may be higher than normal, and the levels may not drop to the normal nighttime low. This will interfere with sleep. If stress continues at high levels, your adrenals can become fatigued and you may develop low cortisol during the day and night. Both scenarios of abnormal cortisol rhythms have health implications and can be associated with sustained pain.

41. Sapolsky, *Why Zebras Don't Get Ulcers*: 64–65, 271–308, 236, 62, 115, 80–81, 152–60.

42. Keith M. Baldwin, "Esophageal Cancer," Medscape Reference, last updated February 4, 2013, http://emedicine.medscape.com/article/277930-overview.

43. M. Pera et al., "Increasing Incidence of Adenocarcinoma of the Esophagus and Esophagogastric Junction," *Gastroenterology* 104, no. 2 (February 1993): 510–13; W. J. Blot et al., "Rising Incidence of Adenocarcinoma of the Esophagus and Gastric Cardia," *Journal of the American Medical Association* 265, no. 10 (March 13, 1991): 1287–89; G. Triadafilopoulos, "Proton Pump Inhibitors for Barrett's Oesophagus," *Gut* 46, no. 2 (February 2000): 144–46.

44. See Yu-Xiao Yang and David C. Metz, "Safety of Proton Pump Inhibitor Exposure," *Gastroenterology* 139, no. 4 (October 2010): 1115–27, www.gastrojournal.org/article/S0016-5085%2810%2901241-2/fulltext, accessed March 12, 2013.

45. E. W. Yu et al., "Acid-Suppressive Medications and Risk of Bone Loss and Fracture in Older Adults," *Calcified Tissue International* 83, no. 4 (October 2008): 251–59.

46. Yang and Metz, "Safety of Proton Pump Inhibitor Exposure."

47. Ibid.

48. B. Golomb and M. Evans, "Statin Adverse Effects: A Review of the Literature and Evidence for a Mitochondrial Mechanism," *American Journal of Cardiovascular Drugs* 8, no. 6 (2009): 373–418.

Chapter 10. Toxic Stew

1. The EPA is the US federal agency charged with protecting Americans from toxins in the environment. In 1998, the agency reported that 43 percent of the twenty-eight hundred chemicals produced in volumes of 1 million pounds per year or more have no basic toxicity data, or screening-level data, at all. Fifty percent have incomplete screening data, and only 7 percent of these so-called high-production-volume (HPV) chemicals have a complete set of screening-level toxicity data. Screening-level data, even if they indicate a problem, are not sufficient to restrict the use of a compound. Summary provided by the Environmental Working Group website: www.chemicalindustryarchives.org/factfiction/facts/1.asp. The origin of the data is the Environmental Protection Agency, Office of Pollution Prevention and Toxics, *Chemical Hazard Data Availability Study: What Do We Really Know about the Safety of High Production Volume Chemicals? EPA's 1998 Baseline of Hazard Information That Is Readily Available to the Public* (Washington, DC: EPA, April 1998), http://www.epa.gov/hpv/pubs/general/hazchem.pdf.

2. D. Davis, *The Secret History of the War on Cancer* (New York: Basic Books, 2007). Devra Davis was the founding director of the Board of Environmental Studies and Toxicology of the National Academy of Sciences and has written extensively on the topic of the consequences of common toxic exposures and how they contribute to our rising cancer rates. She raises the alarm over the unbridled acceptance of chemicals in our environment and the view that the subsequent mortality (deaths) and morbidity (illnesses) are just so much collateral damage on the way of progress. Nena Baker, *The Body Toxic: How the Hazardous Chemistry of Everyday Things Threatens Our Health and Well-Being* (New York: North Point Press, 2008).

3. Environmental Working Group, "Pollution in People: Cord Blood Contaminants in Minority Newborns" (Washington, DC: Environmental Working Group, 2009), http://static.ewg.org/reports/2009/minority_cord_blood/2009-Minority-Cord-Blood-Report.pdf, accessed August 3, 2013. "Summary of Accomplishments," US Environmental Protection Agency website, last updated April 3, 2013, www.epa.gov/oppt/newchems/pubs/accomplishments.htm, accessed June 16, 2013.

4. Environmental Defence, *Polluted Children, Toxic Nation: A Report on Pollution in Canadian Families* (Toronto: Environmental Defence, June 2006), http://environmentaldefence.ca/reports/polluted-children-toxic-nation-report-pollution-canadian-families.

5. M. P. Wilson, D. A. Chia, and B. C. Ehlers, *Green Chemistry in California: A Framework for Leadership in Chemicals Policy and Innovation* (Berkeley: University of California, California Policy Research Center, 2006). The report was prepared for the California Senate Environmental Quality Committee and the California Assembly Committee on Environmental Safety and Toxic Materials.

6. Many toxics are known to be neurotoxic, meaning that they damage or interfere with the function of nerves. This can cause pain. Pain is among the symptoms of lead toxicity listed on the Mayo Clinic website. See "Lead Poisoning," Mayo Clinic, March 12, 2011, www.mayoclinic.com/health/lead-poisoning/FL00068 /DSECTION=symptoms, accessed June 10, 2013.

7. A great book on the devastating, unintended effects of pesticides on the environment and human health is Rachel Carson's *Silent Spring*.

8. Joanne Bradbury, "Docosahexaenoic Acid (DHA): An Ancient Nutrient for the Modern Human Brain," *Nutrients* 3 (2011): 529–54; M. M. Mitchell et al., "Levels of Select PCB and PBDE Congeners in Human Postmortem Brain Reveal Possible Environmental Involvement in 15q11-q13 Duplication Autism Spectrum Disorder," *Environmental and Molecular Mutagenesis* 53, no. 8 (October 2012): 589–98.

9. Environmental Working Group, "Fact #2: People Vary Enormously in Their Reaction to Toxic Substances," Chemical Industry Archives, last updated March 27, 2009, www.chemicalindustryarchives.org/factfiction/facts/2.asp, accessed June 16, 2013.

10. In the United States there is no requirement that genetically modified foods be identified as such. And there is currently a move to put aspartame into flavored milk without including it in the ingredient list.

11. B. Mandelbrot, *The Fractal Geometry of Nature* (New York: W. H. Freeman, 1983).

12. A more complete list of metals: aluminum, antimony, arsenic, barium, beryllium, bismuth, cadmium, cesium, chromium, cobalt, copper, gadolinium, gallium, gold, iron, lead, manganese, mercury, molybdenum, nickel, palladium, platinum, selenium, silver, tellurium, thallium, thorium, tin, titanium, tungsten, uranium, vanadium, and zinc.

13. US Department of Health and Human Services, Public Health Service, and Agency for Toxic Substances and Disease Registry, *Toxicological Profile for Aluminum* (Atlanta: Agency for Toxic Substances and Disease Registry, September 2008), available at www.atsdr.cdc.gov/toxprofiles/tp22.pdf, accessed June 26, 2013. This publication raises the possibility of synergistic effects between aluminum and other heavy metals (p. 204). L. Tomljenovic and C. A. Shaw, "Aluminum Vaccine Adjuvants: Are They Safe?," *Current Medical Chemistry* 18, no. 17 (2011): 2630–37.

14. US Department of Health and Human Services, Public Health Service, and Agency for Toxic Substances and Disease Registry, *Toxicological Profile for Lead* (Atlanta: Agency for Toxic Substances and Disease Registry, August 2007), available at www.atsdr.cdc.gov/toxprofiles/tp13.pdf, accessed June 26, 2013.

15. The chelation challenge is not widely used, but it is discussed in a report published by the US Department of Health and Human Services in 2007. See *Toxicological*

Profile for Lead (Atlanta, GA: US Department of Health and Human Services, Public Health Service, Agency for Toxic Substances and Disease Registry, 2007), www.atsdr.cdc.gov/toxprofiles/tp13.pdf, accessed May 28, 2013.

16. Mark Hyman, "Get This Heavy-Metal Poison Out of Your Body," Dr. Mark Hyman website, May 20, 2010, http://drhyman.com/mercury-get-this-poison -out-of-your-body-85/.

17. K. M. Cecil et al., "Decreased Brain Volume in Adults with Childhood Lead Exposure," *PLoS Medicine* 5, no. 5 (2008); J. P. Wright et al., "Association of Prenatal and Childhood Blood Lead Concentrations with Criminal Arrests in Early Adulthood," *PLoS Medicine* 5, no. 5 (2008): 732–39; D. C. Bellinger, "Neurological and Behavioral Consequences of Childhood Lead Exposure," *PLoS Medicine* 5, no. 5 (2008).

18. A. Menke et al., "Blood Lead Below 0.48 μmol/L (10 μg/dL) and Mortality among US Adults," *Circulation* 114, no. 13 (September 26, 2006): 1388–94.

19. Jonathan J. Carmouche et al., "Lead Exposure Inhibits Fracture Healing and Is Associated with Increased Chondrogenesis, Delay in Cartilage Mineralization, and a Decrease in Osteoprogenitor Frequency," *Environmental Health Perspectives* 113 (2005): 749–55; Joel G. Pounds, Gregory J. Long, and John F. Rosen, "Cellular and Molecular Toxicity of Lead in Bone," *Environmental Health Perspectives* 91 (1991): 17–32.

20. A. Rowland and R. McKinstry, "Lead Toxicity, White Matter Lesions, and Aging," *Neurology* 66, no. 10 (May 2006): 1464–65.

21. Wendy McKelvey et al., "A Biomonitoring Study of Lead, Cadmium and Mercury in the Blood of New York City Adults," *Environmental Health Perspectives* 115, no. 10 (October 2007): 1435–41.

22. D. Cole et al., "Environmental Contaminant Levels and Fecundability among Non-smoking Couples," *Reproductive Toxicology* 22, no. 1 (July 2006): 13–19.

23. This occurs through the release of an inflammatory mediator from a class of human immune cells called mast cells.

24. "Thimerosal in Vaccines," US Food and Drug Administration, last updated June 6, 2012, www.fda.gov/BiologicsBloodVaccines/SafetyAvailability/Vaccine -Safety/UCM096228#t3, accessed June 26, 2013.

25. T. Wanga et al., "Total Phenolic Compounds, Radical Scavenging and Metal Chelation of Extracts from Icelandic Seaweeds," *Food Chemistry* 116, no. 1 (September 2009): 240–48.

26. "Information Sheet: Pharmaceuticals in Drinking-Water," World Health Organization, undated, www.who.int/water_sanitation_health/emerging/info_sheet _pharmaceuticals/en/index.html, accessed June 16, 2013.

27. According to the October 17, 2007, issue of the *Journal of the American Medical Association*, methicillin-resistant *Staphylococcus aureus* alone is now responsible for an estimated 94,000 life-threatening infections and 18,650 deaths (R. M. Klevens

et al., "Invasive Methicillin-Resistant *Staphylococcus Aureus* Infections in the United States," *Journal of the American Medical Association* 298, no. 15 [2007]: 1763–71). An estimated 73,480 illnesses due to *E. coli* O157 infection occur each year in the United States, leading to an estimated 2,168 hospitalizations and 61 deaths annually, and it is an important cause of acute renal failure in children (Josefa M. Rangel, "Epidemiology of *Escherichia coli* O157:H7 Outbreaks, United States, 1982–2002," *Journal of Emerging Infectious Diseases* 11, no. 4 [April 2005], CDC website, wwwnc.cdc.gov/eid/article/11/4/04-0739_article.htm, accessed April 18, 2013).

28. J. S. de Vendomois et al., "A Comparison of the Effects of Three GM Corn Varieties on Mammalian Health," *International Journal of Biological Sciences* 5, no. 7 (2009): 706–26.

29. R. S. Gupta et al., "The Prevalence, Severity, and Distribution of Childhood Food Allergy in the United States," *Pediatrics* 128, no. 1 (2011): 9–17.

30. Leif G. Salford et al., "Téléphonie mobile et barrière sang-cerveau," in *Téléphonie Mobile — Effets Potentiels sur la Santé des Ondes Électromagnétiques de Haute Fréquence*, ed. Pietteur Marco (Embourg, Belgium: Collection Resurgence, 2001), 141–52.

31. Leif G. Salford et al., "Nerve Cell Damage in Mammalian Brain after Exposure to Microwaves from GSM Mobile Phones," *Environmental Health Perspectives* 111, no. 7 (June 2003): 881–83.

32. As we saw earlier, heavy metals are also neurotoxic.

33. *Environmental Threats to Children's Health in America's Schools: The Case for Prevention: Before the Comm. on Environment and Public Works*, 107th Cong. (2002) (testimony of Philip J. Landrigan, MD, MSc, director of the Center for Children's Health and the Environment at Mount Sinai School of Medicine, New York, NY). www.epw.senate.gov/107th/Landrigan_100102.htm.

Chapter 11. Your Team

1. H. Green et al., "Impaired Sarcoplasmic Reticulum Calcium Adenosine Triphosphate Expression and Function in Work-Induced Myalgia," unpublished manuscript.

2. J. Achterberg et al., "Evidence for Correlations between Distant Intentionality and Brain Function in Recipients: A Functional Magnetic Resonance Imaging Analysis," *Journal of Alternative and Complementary Medicine* 11, no. 6 (2005): 965–71.

3. S. A. Skootsky, B. Jaeger, and R. K. Oye, "Prevalence of Myofascial Pain in General Internal Medicine Practice," *Western Journal of Medicine* 151, no. 2 (1989): 157–60. Skootsky, Jaeger, and Oye found that 30 percent of regular patients in a general medical clinic met criteria for MFPS. S. Marklund and A. Wänman, "Incidence and Prevalence of Myofascial Pain in the Jaw-Face Region: A One-Year

Prospective Study on Dental Students," *Acta Odontologica Scandinavica* 66, no. 2 (2008): 113–21. Marklund and Wänman found that 19 percent of normal dental students develop MFPS over a year. S. Roach et al., "Prevalence of Myofascial Trigger Points in the Hip in Patellofemoral Pain," *Archives of Physical Medicine and Rehabilitation* 94, no. 3 (2013): 522–26. Roach et al. found that approximately 90 percent of patients with patellofemoral pain had MF trigger points, and 30 percent of normal controls did. David G. Simons, "Clinical and Etiological Update of Myofascial Pain from Trigger Points," *Journal of Musculoskeletal Pain* 4, no. 1–2 (1996): 1–2. According to Simons, between 30 and 93 percent of patients with pain anywhere in the body had myofascial trigger points.

4. Z. H. Cho et al., "New Findings of the Correlation between Acupoints and Corresponding Brain Cortices Using Functional MRI," *Proceedings of the National Academy of Sciences USA* 95, no. 5 (March 3, 1998): 2670–73.

5. World Health Organization, *Acupuncture: Review and Analysis of Reports on Controlled Clinical Trials* (Geneva: WHO, 2003), http://apps.who.int/medicine docs/pdf/s4926e/s4926e.pdf, accessed June 13, 2013.

6. "Acupuncture for Pain," National Center for Complementary and Alternative Medicine, last updated August 2010, http://nccam.nih.gov/health/acupuncture /acupuncture-for-pain.htm?nav=gsa, accessed June 13, 2013.

7. C. Chan Gunn, MD, *The Gunn Approach to the Treatment of Chronic Pain: Intramuscular Stimulation for Myofascial Pain of Radiculopathic Origin* (New York: Churchill Livingstone, 1996).

8. "There is little doubt that root compression lesions from discogenic disease are one of the most common maladies of bipedal man." J. Goodgold and A. Eberstein, *Electrodiagnosis of Neuromuscular Diseases*, 2nd ed. (Baltimore: Williams and Wilkins, 1983).

9. W. B. Cannon and A. Rosenbluth, *The Supersensitivity of Denervated Structures* (New York: Macmillan, 1949).

10. There are over two hundred different systems of techniques for manipulation. Jay Triano DC, PhD, dean of Graduate Education and Research, Canadian Memorial Chiropractic College, personal communication, June 2010.

11. J. J. Triano et al., "Inner Psoas Tri-axial Deformation under Tensile Load Corresponds to Superficial Dense Connective Tissue Morphology," in *Fascia Research II, Basic Science and Implications for Conventional and Complementary Health Care*, ed. P. A. Huijing et al. (Munich: Elsevier, 2009), 216.

12. The work of Vladimir Janda, a neurologist and physiatrist in Czechoslovakia, also foreshadowed the later discoveries about fascia. Janda showed that patients who had an imbalance in the tone of some of their muscle groups had predictable patterns of pain and dysfunction. He also showed that we are programmed to learn

certain skills in particular postures. For example, babies learn to use alternate arm and leg movements when they crawl. He developed a program of progressive exercises that challenged patients' balance and position to improve posture, muscle balance, and joint stability. His therapies addressed how structure and function, and musculoskeletal and neurological systems, entwined in an ongoing dance of compensation and adaptation as the body strives toward equilibrium. There is an amusing depiction of the work of Rolf and Janda in the 1977 movie *Semi-tough*, with football team owner Robert Preston crawling around his office floor and sending his toughest player for Rolfing sessions.

13. C. Ober, S. Sinatra, and M. Zucker, *Earthing: The Most Important Health Discovery Ever?* (Laguna Beach, CA: Basic Health Publications, 2010).

14. There is a controversy about whether Reiki is a new or rediscovered treatment.

15. I find that taping an ankle is more effective that a stretchy bandage. The tape better supports the sprained ligaments and does not fully encircle the ankle, so it does not cut off circulation.

16. Russell Jaffe, *Health Studies Collegium Handbook* (Reston, VA: Serammune Physicians Laboratories, 1987), appendix 8, p. 30.

17. Normally light radiates out in all directions from its source and is made up of many different wavelengths. Laser light, however, is coherent, meaning there is a single wavelength and all the light waves line up and travel in the same direction: there is very little scatter of the light. Cold laser can use light-emitting diodes in clusters or single diode units of higher energy.

18. C. Vallbona et al., "Response of Pain to Static Magnetic Fields in Postpolio Patients: A Double-Blind Pilot Study," *Archives of Physical Medicine and Rehabilitation* 78, no. 11 (November 1997): 1200–1203.

19. "Although the present review does not provide proof of efficacy for any individual technique, it clearly shows that no difference exists between trigger point injections with different substances, or between dry and wet needling." T. M. Cummings et al., "Needling Therapies in the Management of Myofascial Trigger Point Pain: A Systematic Review," *Archives of Physical Medicine and Rehabilitation* 82, no. 7 (2001): 986–92, www.sciencedirect.com/science/article/pii/S0003999301066564, accessed April 27, 2013.

20. T. A. Garvey, M. R. Marks, and S. W. Wiesel, "A Prospective, Randomized, Double-Blind Evaluation of Trigger-Point Injection Therapy for Low-Back Pain," *Spine* 14, no. 9 (1989): 962–64.

21. Some stroke patients develop contracted muscles on the side of the body affected by the damage to the brain.

22. J. Buric, "Chemyonucleolysis vs Microdiscectomy Prospective Controlled Study with 18 Months' Follow-Up," *Rivista Italiana di Ossigeno-Ozonoterapia* 4 (2005): 49–54.

23. H. A. Wilkinson, "Injection Therapy for Enthesopathies Causing Axial Spine Pain and the "Failed Back Syndrome": A Single-Blinded, Randomized and Crossover Study" *Pain Physician* 8, no. 2 (April 2005): 167–73.

24. A. Mishra, J. Woodall Jr., and A. Vieira, "Treatment of Tendon and Muscle Using Platelet-Rich Plasma," *Clinics in Sports Medicine* 28, no. 1 (January 2009): 113–25.

25. J. Loeser, "Other Surgical Interventions," *Pain Practice* 6, no. 1 (March 2006): 59.

26. W. A. Macrae, "Chronic Pain after Surgery," *British Journal of Anaesthesia* 87, no. 1 (2001): 88–98. This article is a review of many studies on chronic pain after common surgeries.

27. J. D. Loeser, "The Role of the Multidisciplinary Pain Clinic," in *Surgical Management of Pain*, ed. K. J. Burchiel (New York: Thieme Medical Publishers, 2002), 237–45.

28. H. A. Wilkinson, *The Failed Back Syndrome: Etiology and Therapy*, 2nd ed. (Philadelphia: Harper and Row, 1991).

Chapter 12. The Road to Recovery

1. The Arizona Center for Integrative Medicine, at the University of Arizona, is the educational organization established by Andrew Weil to teach integrative medicine to physicians.

Glossary

1. Institute for Functional Medicine website, 2013, www.functionalmedicine.org/.

2. "About Holistic Medicine: What Is Holistic Medicine?," American Holistic Medical Association website, undated, www.holisticmedicine.org/content .asp?pl=2&sl=43&contentid=43.

3. National Center for Homeopathy website, 2013, http://nationalcenterfor homeopathy.org/.

GLOSSARY

ACTH (adrenocorticotropic hormone): A hormone produced in and secreted by the anterior pituitary gland. It causes an increase in corticosteroid production and release. Corticosteroids reduce inflammation.

Acupuncture: The use of very fine needles to stimulate energy pathways in the body called meridians. Acupuncture is part of an ancient system of medicine developed in China called Traditional Chinese Medicine.

Acute pain: Pain that lasts less than six months.

Adaptogen: A substance used in natural medicine to decrease the body's response to stress.

Adrenal glands: Glands located above the kidneys that release hormones as a response to stress.

Adrenaline: Also known as epinephrine, a stress hormone produced by the adrenal glands.

Alexander technique: A method of teaching movement awareness to help people move more freely and in a more relaxed and comfortable way by changing harmful habits.

Allodynia: Experiencing pain from nonpainful stimuli. (See related *hyperalgesia*.)

Allopathic medicine: The "conventional" medicine taught to doctors in our current medical school system. Allopathic medicine usually involves tests, drugs, and procedures and is most concerned with treating disease that is already established.

Alpha-linolenic acid: An omega-3 fatty acid that reduces inflammation in the body. It is an essential nutrient, meaning humans cannot make it and must consume some of it.

Amygdala: Part of the brain that plays a role in emotional memory, especially fear.

Anabolic steroids: Drugs that have an effect similar to that of testosterone.

Analgesics: Painkillers.

Anti-inflammatory: A class of drugs designed to reduce inflammation. (See *nonsteroidal anti-inflammatories [NSAIDs]*.)

Antioxidant: Helpful molecules that reduce and repair damage to our tissues and cells that can be caused by oxidative stress.

Arthroscope: A medical device used to do surgery on joints through tiny incisions.

Ashwagandha: A specific herb that helps the body deal with stress.

Autoimmune disorder (autoimmunity): A condition in which the body's immune system attacks its own tissues. This can cause pain, inflammation, and disease.

Autonomic nervous system: The autonomic system is part of our nervous system, and it has two parts, called the sympathetic and parasympathetic systems. These regulate functions we regard as automatic, like blood pressure control, heart rate, breathing, bowel function, and others.

Ayurveda: An ancient system of healing developed in India.

Blood-brain barrier: System that creates a protective barrier around the brain and prevents many of the things circulating through the body from reaching and damaging the brain.

Botulinum toxin: An injectable substance derived from a toxin produced by bacteria. It is used to block signals from the nerves to the muscles.

Bursa: A small structure that is present around some joints and that allows muscles and tendons to slide smoothly over each other during movement.

Bursitis: Inflammation of a bursa.

Carpal tunnel: A half-inch area on the inside of the wrist where nine tendons and the median nerve pass from the wrist into the hand.

Carpal tunnel syndrome: Excessive pressure on the median nerve as it passes through a small space in the wrist. Carpal tunnel syndrome may cause numbness and tingling in the thumb, the index finger, the middle finger, and half of the ring finger.

Catechin: An antioxidant and natural phenol found in tea, chocolate, and red wine.

Catecholamines: Neurotransmitters that are involved in our stress responses. Two of them are adrenaline and noradrenaline, which are also called epinephrine and norepinephrine.

Celiac disease: A genetic sensitivity to gluten. Some people with celiac disease show signs of it in early childhood, while others seem to develop it in adulthood. Most people with celiac disease have bowel symptoms such as severe diarrhea with bowel damage. Celiac disease can also be associated with pain anywhere in the body. Celiac disease and gluten intolerance are two different conditions that can affect people who are genetically predisposed toward them. (See also *gluten intolerance.*)

Chelation: This is a chemical process in which an organic compound (that is, a compound containing carbon) attaches to metals. Medically this process is used to treat heavy-metal poisoning, such as by lead or mercury, and sometimes is used in treating heart disease.

Chiropractic medicine: A form of complementary and alternative medicine that involves manual manipulation of the spine and other joints.

Chronic fatigue and immune deficiency syndrome (CFIDS): A poorly understood condition that causes fatigue, pain, and some abnormalities of the immune system. It likely has many different causes, which may include infections, exposures to toxics, food intolerances, excessive stress, allergies, and others. It is sometimes called chronic fatigue.

Chronic pain: Pain that lasts longer than six months (some authorities define it as longer than three months).

Chronic regional pain syndrome (CRPS): Chronic pain that is usually caused by some form of nerve damage. Often the pain is described as burning or shooting.

Cofactors: Micronutrients that help the body's metabolism.

Cognitive behavioral therapy (CBT): A form of psychotherapy that focuses on changing behavior by increasing awareness of inaccurate or negative thinking.

Collagen: A protein crucial to the formation of connective tissue.

Complementary and alternative medicine (CAM): *Alternative medicine* is the label given to anything other than what is done by allopathically trained doctors (that is, those trained in conventional medical schools). It includes acupuncture, massage, chiropractic, osteopathy, and herbal medicine. *Complementary medicine* refers to treatments that are outside allopathic medicine that would be used along with conventional medicine.

Craniosacral therapy: A very gentle technique used to relieve tightness in deep structures of the body.

Cryoablation: Freezing nerves to treat nerve pain.

Cytotoxic: Deadly to cells.

de Quervain's tenosynovitis: Painful inflammation of the tendons located at the sides of the thumb caused by overuse of the thumb. It is a myofascial condition of tight muscles above the wrist.

Dermatitis: A scaly and/or itchy condition of the skin caused by inflammation. There are many different causes.

Diabetes: A condition of high blood glucose and insulin resistance. Type I diabetes always requires insulin and usually develops in children. Type II usually develops later in life and is associated with obesity. Type II can initially be managed by exercise and diet.

Dichlorodiphenyltrichloroethane (DDT): A highly toxic pesticide banned in the United States since 1972.

Dioxins: A family of highly toxic chemicals that are mostly the result of industrial processes. They are part of the "dirty dozen," a group of dangerous chemicals known as persistent organic pollutants.

Diverticulum: An abnormal outpouching in the body. Diverticula can occur in the bowel; if they become inflamed, this is called diverticulitis.

Docosahexaenoic acid (DHA): Omega-3 fatty acid found in fish oil and algae. Especially good for the brain.

Dualism: Any theory or philosophy that suggests the mind is separate from the body.

Dysbiosis: An imbalance of microbes in the body.

Dysesthesia: Impaired sensation.

Eczema: A common term for dermatitis, or inflammation of the skin. Symptoms include dryness, itching, redness, and swelling of the skin.

Eicosapentaenoic acid (EPA): An omega-3 fatty acid found in fish oil.

Elimination diet: Method of identifying food allergies by systematically eliminating foods from one's diet.

Endocrine system: A network of glands that secrete hormones into the bloodstream. These hormones regulate growth, metabolism, and sexual development.

Endorphins: Naturally occurring opioids, or painkillers, made by the brain and nervous system

Epinephrine: Also known as adrenaline, a stress hormone produced by the adrenal glands.

Essential nutrients: Those nutrients that humans cannot produce and must therefore get from their diet.

Fascia: A layer of connective tissue that covers and connects body structures, including muscles, muscle groups, nerves, and blood vessels. It is a body-wide communication system.

Fatty liver: A condition in which fat accumulates in the liver. This can be due to alcoholism or poor diet. It has also been associated with the consumption of high-fructose corn syrup.

Feldenkrais method: A way of teaching movement awareness to help people reconnect with their natural ability to move, think, and feel. The lessons are designed to improve everyday function.

Fibromyalgia: The painful condition generally defined by a sleep disorder and excess tenderness of at least eleven of eighteen specific points that have been mapped out on the body. People with fibromyalgia have upper- and lower-body pain, and right- and left-side pain. The causes are unknown. This definition was developed to help group people together for studies of the condition. Fibromyalgia is associated with changes in the central nervous system that cause people to be hypersensitive to pain.

Fluoroscope: A tool that uses X-rays to examine the inner structures of the body.

Free radicals: High-energy particles that can damage our cells. Some free radicals are produced by the body during normal metabolism, and some come from the external environment.

Functional medicine: Defined by the Institute for Functional Medicine as addressing the "underlying causes of disease, using a systems-oriented approach and engaging both patient and practitioner in a therapeutic partnership."[1]

Gamma-linolenic acid (GLA): An omega-6 fatty acid that is found in vegetable oils.

Ganglion cyst: A fluid-filled outpouching on a tendon caused by overuse and usually associated with myofascial tightness of the associated muscles.

Gangrene: A condition in which restricted blood flow and infection cause body tissue to die.

Gastroesophageal reflux disease (GERD): A condition in which acid flows upward from the stomach into the swallowing tube called the esophagus. A cause of heartburn.

Gene expression: How or even whether the information from a gene gets used. For example, not everyone with the genes for heart disease will get heart disease. A heart-healthy lifestyle may keep those genes from being expressed.

Giant cell arteritis: An inflammatory condition of the vessels in the scalp, neck, and arms that causes the vessels to narrow and restrict blood flow.

Gluten intolerance: A genetic sensitivity to gluten that usually does not cause severe diarrhea. Often there are skin irritations associated with gluten intolerance. It can also be associated with ill health and pain anywhere in the body.

Gunn IMS: A treatment for myofascial pain based on the theories of Chan Gunn. Acupuncture needles are used to treat trigger points and the muscles close to the spine. Gunn IMS is similar to dry needling and intramuscular stimulation (IMS), but Gunn IMS incorporates physical examination and additional treatment to address the dysfunction of the nerves that is associated with the development of persistent trigger points.

Hemochromatosis: A genetic disorder causing the body to store iron inappropriately.

Hemoglobin: A protein in red blood cells that carries oxygen to cells.

Herniated disc: A common condition that happens when there is damage to the disc that normally creates a cushion between the vertebral bones of the spine. It may also be called a slipped or bulging disc. The contents of the disc protrude and sometimes cause pain, but often the condition is painless. Usually happens in the lower back or neck.

High-fructose corn syrup: A sweetener made from corn and added to many processed foods. It converts quickly into fat and is associated with fatty liver.

Hippocampus: The part of the brain responsible for memory and spatial navigation.

Holistic medicine: The American Holistic Medical Association defines holistic medicine as "the art and science of healing that addresses care of the whole person — body, mind, and spirit."[2]

Homeopathy: The National Center for Homeopathy describes homeopathy as a "form of natural medicine that works to heal the body rather than simply treat an illness's symptoms."[3]

Homeostatic: Characterized by homeostasis, the body's natural tendency to move toward a state of balance.

Homocysteine: A naturally occurring amino acid in the blood. High levels of it may indicate problems with the metabolic step called methylation.

Hydrogenated oils: Oils that have been altered to give them a different texture.

Hyperalgesia: Experiencing excess pain from a mildly uncomfortable stimulus. (See related *allodynia*.)

Insulin resistance: A condition in which the cells of the body do not respond normally to insulin. It is associated with type 2 diabetes.

Integrative medicine: The latest in the terms used to describe the integrated use of multidisciplinary teams to prevent illness and treat disease. This approach to medicine is patient centered, focuses on prevention, and pays attention to mind, body, and spirit. It makes use of all appropriate approaches and disciplines to provide the best treatment for the patient.

Interstitial cystitis: A chronic condition characterized by bladder pain.

Intervertebral discs: Small structures that act like cushions between the vertebrae, or spinal bones.

Intramuscular stimulation (IMS): Also called dry needling. A technique using acupuncture needles or empty hypodermic needles to stimulate myofascial trigger points.

Laban-Bartenieff work: A method of teaching movement awareness that has its origins in dance. It teaches a way to understand and explore movement.

Laser therapy: The use of low-intensity medical laser light to put energy into tissues and stimulate healing. Such lasers are sometimes called cold lasers to distinguish them from the cutting or burning lasers used in surgery.

Leptin: A hormone that influences food consumption and energy expenditure.

Linoleic acid: A type of omega-6 fatty acid that, in the Western diet, is usually eaten in high amounts. It promotes inflammation when eaten in excess. It is an essential nutrient, meaning humans cannot make it and must consume some of it.

Lipid peroxidation: Damage caused by free radicals to the polyunsaturated fatty acids in the cell membranes.

Lipids: Compounds that are fatty acids or derived from fatty acids. They do not dissolve in water. These are especially important for our cell membranes and our brain.

Lipophilic: Attracted to and able to dissolve in lipids.

Lymphocytes: White blood cells; part of the immune system.

Lymphoma: A blood cancer that occurs in lymphocytes.

Matcha: A high-quality green tea sold in leaf or powdered form. Considerable research has shown that matcha is useful for Alzheimer's prevention.

Melatonin: A hormone produced by the pineal gland that promotes a good night's sleep. It is also a powerful antioxidant.

Metabolite: A substance produced when a foreign or naturally occurring chemical or a drug is processed by the metabolic system.

Microbes: Tiny organisms called microorganisms, such as bacteria, viruses, yeasts, protozoa, parasites, and others.

Microbiome: The mass of microorganisms in the gut, mouth, skin, vagina, and lungs. In the gut the microbiome helps us digest and absorb our food and keeps our immune system healthy.

Microcurrent: A form of electrical stimulation that uses microamp electrical current.

Microdistilled: Purification process used for producing uncontaminated fish oils.

Microglial cells: Immune-system housekeeping cells in the brain and spinal cord. They heal the nerve cells but may also cause damage to them under certain circumstances.

Mind-body medicine: The growing field of medicine that treats the whole person and takes into account physical, psychological, and spiritual aspects. It recognizes the interconnectedness of all the body systems.

Mitochondria: Energy-producing parts of cells.

Monocytes: Immune system cells involved in immune function and inflammation.

Monounsaturated oils: Fats that contain one double bond.

Movement therapies: There are several schools of movement therapy, and all take the student back to an awareness of more efficient and basic patterns of movement as a means of restoring health.

Myofascial: A condition of overtight muscles and fascia (the supporting connective tissues) that is a common cause of musculoskeletal pain. Treatment usually involves releasing trigger points in muscles.

Naturopathy: A system of natural medicine that focuses on the body's own ability to heal.

Nerve conduction test: A medical test to see how fast electrical current passes along a nerve. Results may be normal even when there is subtle damage in or dysfunction of a nerve, as long as the nerve is not yet dying.

Neuropathic: Dysfunction of a nerve.

Neuroplasticity: The ability of the nervous system to change itself.

Neurotoxin: Anything that is toxic to nerves.

Nonsteroidal anti-inflammatories (NSAIDs): Anti-inflammatories that are not steroids; they are pain relievers.

Noradrenaline: Also known as norepinephrine, a stress hormone produced by the adrenal glands.

Norepinephrine: Also known as noradrenaline, a stress hormone produced by the adrenal glands.

Nutrigenomics: How food affects our gene expression.

Omega-3 fatty acids: Polyunsaturated fatty acids found in foods such as fish and flaxseed. In proper amounts they can help to decrease inflammation.

Osteoarthritis: Wear-and-tear arthritis. Associated with reduced thickness of the cartilage that cushions the joints.

Osteonecrosis: Death of bone.

Osteopathy: A holistic system of medicine that emphasizes the interrelation of the structure and functions of the body.

Osteopenia: Bone density that is lower than normal but not low enough to be classified as osteoporosis.

Osteoporosis: Low bone density, which makes bones more likely to fracture.

Oxidative stress: Damage done by free radicals. It can be neutralized by antioxidants. Oxidative stress is involved in many degenerative diseases, such as atherosclerosis, and is associated with aging.

Oxytocin: A feel-good hormone that is elevated when we hug or kiss a loved one. Levels also go up during sex, birth, and breast-feeding.

Parabens: Chemicals used as preservatives in cosmetics and pharmaceuticals. Parabens may have harmful effects on the body and interfere with hormones.

Parasympathetic nervous system: The part of the autonomic nervous system that is responsible for the normal functioning of many of our internal organ systems. It is designed to be in balance with the sympathetic nervous system. It dominates when we are in a relaxed state.

Petrochemicals: Chemicals made from petroleum.

Phthalates: Chemicals found in cosmetics that may have harmful effects on the body and interfere with hormones.

Physiological dose: Dose of a hormone that is the same as a healthy body would make.

Phytochemicals: Naturally occurring chemicals found in plants or derived from them.

Pineal gland: A tiny gland in the brain that makes melatonin and other hormones.

Piriformis syndrome: A syndrome caused by tightness of the piriformis muscle, which is deep in the buttock. This muscle lies in very close contact with the sciatic nerve and can cause pressure on that nerve, resulting in sciatica. Piriformis syndrome can mimic a herniated disc in the lumbar spine.

Polychlorinated biphenyl (PCB): A toxic pollutant that can become concentrated in our tissues.

Polyphenols: A large family of health-beneficial, natural compounds from plants.

Polyunsaturated fatty acids (PUFA): Healthy fats that contain more than one double bond.

Prebiotics: Nutrients that help probiotics to thrive in the gut.

Premenstrual syndrome: A collection of symptoms that occur before the menstrual period, including bloating, weight gain, breast pain, acne, and mood changes.

Probiotics: Bacteria in the gut that are essential for proper gut function.

Prolotherapy: An injection technique to tighten ligaments and tendons.

Prostaglandins: Chemical messengers within cells. They can both promote and resolve inflammation.

Psyllium husks: A good source of fiber, especially if natural and unsweetened.

Quercetin: A flavonoid antioxidant present in many plants.

Qi gong: A moving meditation that integrates breathing, movement, and exercise to move chi, or life-force energy, within the body.

Radio-frequency ablation: A technique to burn structures, such as nerves, in an attempt to reduce pain. The nerves regrow over time.

Raynaud disease: A condition in which blood vessels narrow in reaction to cold or other stressors. The fingers, toes, nose, and ears are commonly affected, and they can turn blue or white and feel numb and cold. It is more common among women and in colder climates.

Reflex sympathetic dystrophy: An older name for chronic regional pain syndrome.

Reiki: A technique for stress reduction and relaxation that originated in Japan. It is a healing practice in which the practitioner uses his or her hands to pass healing energy to the patient.

Repetitive strain injury (RSI): An injury that occurs when most of the body is in a static posture and a few parts of the body are used to do the same or similar activities repeatedly.

Resveratrol: A powerful antioxidant from grapes, wine, peanuts, and some berries.

Reverse osmosis: A water-purification technique using a semipermeable membrane.

Rhabdomyolysis: The breakdown of muscles, causing muscle fiber contents to leak into the bloodstream and cause kidney damage.

Rheumatoid arthritis: A chronic autoimmune disorder that causes inflammation of the joints and surrounding tissues.

Rhodiola: The extract of the plant *Rhodiola rosea*, traditionally used to prevent fatigue and enhance physical and mental performance. It is an adaptogen.

Rickets: A weakening of the bones of children, causing the legs to bow. Produced by vitamin D deficiency.

Rotator cuff dysfunction: A common condition in which the muscles around the shoulder are injured, weak, or damaged. Inflammation is often not a major factor.

Rotator cuff tendinitis: Inflammation of the tendons of the muscles around the shoulder blade.

Sciatica: Pain down the back or side of the thigh and leg caused by pressure on the nerves of the low back. It is commonly thought to be caused by pressure from the intervertebral discs, but recent studies have confirmed that piriformis syndrome is more common.

Serotonin: A hormone and neurotransmitter that regulates mood, appetite, and sleep. Eighty percent of the body's serotonin production occurs in the gut.

Silymarin: An extract of milk thistle or certain other plants. Silymarin helps the liver enzymes detoxify substances and helps protect the liver.

Somatic nervous system: The part of the nervous system that controls our voluntary movements.

Spelt: A nutritious and ancient grain similar to wheat. Spelt contains gluten.

Statins: Substances that interfere with the cells' ability to produce cholesterol.

Steroid: An anti-inflammatory drug that mimics the cortisol from our adrenal glands.

Stevia: A sweetener extracted from the leaf of a plant. It is three hundred times as sweet as sugar and has a negligible effect on blood glucose.

Sucralose: An artificial sweetener made from sugar and chlorine that is six hundred times as sweet as sugar.

Sympathetic nervous system: Part of the autonomic nervous system responsible for the fight-or-flight reaction. The sympathetic nervous system gets overstimulated when a person is anxious.

Sympathectomy: The surgical cutting or removal of sympathetic nerves in an attempt to decrease pain.

Tai chi: An ancient Chinese martial art that is also a moving meditation. Its movements are useful for enhancing balance, coordination, and strength, and for reducing painful conditions.

Telomeres: The ends of DNA strands that protect the DNA from damage. They act like the ends of our shoelaces (aglets), which keep the laces from unraveling. Telomeres enable our chromosomes to divide to make new cells. Age and chronic stress shorten telomeres. Proper telomere length is associated with longevity.

Tendinitis: Inflammation of tendons.

Tendinosis: Damage to the tendons.

Tendon: The connective tissue that attaches muscle to bone.

Tenosynovitis: Inflammation around a tendon that has an extra layer of connective tissue called a synovium.

Thoracic outlet: The location at the side of the neck in which the veins, arteries, and nerves pass through a small area.

Thoracic outlet syndrome: Compression of the veins, arteries, and nerves as they pass through the thoracic outlet. It is often caused by myofascial muscle tightness. There may also be extra connective tissue bands or an extra cervical rib that can cause compression in the area.

Thyroid: The endocrine gland at the base of the neck, responsible for metabolism regulation.

Tocopherols: Parts of the vitamin E family. All are antioxidants. There are four tocopherols (alpha, beta, gamma, and delta). Alpha is the most readily absorbed by the body. Much of the vitamin E on the market is synthetic alpha-tocopherol, which may have less therapeutic value than natural vitamin E, which has all eight parts.

Tocotrienols: Parts of the vitamin E family. There are four kinds.

Traditional Chinese Medicine: A range of therapies developed in China, including acupuncture, herbal medicine, massage (tui na), exercise (qi gong), and diet.

Trager movement education: An approach to movement education that involves two components. One is table work, in which a trained practitioner uses movements and touch to help release deep-seated patterns that may contribute to ill health or pain. The second component involves self-movements that enable greater freedom of movement and repatterning.

Transcutaneous electrical nerve stimulator (TENS): A small device used to treat pain by means of electricity applied through gel pads.

Trans fats: Processed fats chemically modified to change the consistency and increase the shelf life of food. Consumption of trans fats increases the risk of heart disease and stroke.

Traumeel: A homeopathic pain reliever that can be applied to the skin or taken as a homeopathic pill.

Trigger finger: A painful condition characterized by either the catching or the locking of a finger in a bent position. It is often caused by a nodule on the tendon that gets stuck in the pulley system that controls the movement of the tendons.

Trigger points (TPs): Overcontracted, supersensitive injured areas of muscle that are often associated with pain.

Trigger point massage: A technique using very firm pressure in order to release TPs.

Turmeric/curcumin: Curcumin is the primary constituent in turmeric, a spice that is an anti-inflammatory and a pain reliever.

Ulcerative colitis: A type of inflammatory bowel disease that causes ulcers in the lining of the colon and rectum.

Uric acids: Chemicals created when the body breaks down certain foods, especially meat products. Uric acid usually travels in the blood to the kidneys and is excreted in the urine. Abnormally high amounts of uric acid can be due to alcoholism, diabetes, or the consumption of too much fructose. Uric-acid crystal deposits cause gout.

Vasoconstriction: Constriction or tightening of the muscles of blood vessels. This can cause poor circulation or high blood pressure. It can be a factor in pain.

Vasodilatation: Dilation or relaxation of the muscles of blood vessels. Warm temperatures and relaxation cause healthy levels of vasodilation.

Xenoestrogens: Artificial chemicals in plastics, cosmetics, and pesticides that act like powerful estrogens once they are in the body.

Xylitol: An artificial sweetener with two-thirds the calories of sugar. Considered safe for diabetics. May have some protective value for dental enamel.

Yoga: An ancient practice of movements and breathing techniques. It is a moving meditation.

RESOURCES

This list contains readings, CDs, DVDs, and websites you may find helpful. It is not an exhaustive list. I am not endorsing or necessarily agreeing with everything said in each one, but all can help you educate yourself about nutrition, health, pain, and integrative medicine.

Chronic Pain

Caudill, M. *Managing Pain before It Manages You.* 3rd ed. Guilford Press, 2008.

Cohen, D. *Turning Suffering Inside Out: A Zen Approach to Living with Physical and Emotional Pain.* Shambhala, 2002.

Turk, D., and F. Winter. *The Pain Survival Guide: How to Reclaim Your Life.* American Psychological Association, 2005.

Integrative Health

Blanchard, K., and M. A. Brill. *What Your Doctor May Not Tell You about Hypothyroidism: A Simple Plan for Extraordinary Results.* Warner Books, 2004.

Gibson, R., and J. P. Singh. *The Treatment Trap: How the Overuse of Medical Care Is Wrecking Your Health, and What You Can Do to Prevent It.* Rowman and Littlefield, 2011.

Lee, J., and V. Hopkins. *What Your Doctor May Not Tell You about Menopause: The Breakthrough Book on Natural Hormone Balance.* Warner Books, 2004.

Northrup, C. *Women's Bodies, Women's Wisdom: Creating Physical and Emotional Health and Healing.* Bantam, 2001.

Ornish, D. *Dr. Dean Ornish's Program for Reversing Heart Disease: The Only System Scientifically Proven to Reverse Heart Disease without Drugs or Surgery.* Random House, 1990.

Roizen, M., and M. Oz. *You — The Owner's Manual: An Insider's Guide to the Body That Will Make You Healthier and Younger.* HarperCollins, 2005.

Weil, A. *Natural Health, Natural Medicine: The Complete Guide to Wellness and Self-Care for Optimum Health.* Houghton Mifflin, 1995.

Escape Fire: The Fight to Rescue American Healthcare (DVD). Directed by Susan Frömke and Matthew Heineman, 2012.

Nutrition

Campbell-McBride, N. *Gut and Psychology Syndrome: Natural Treatment for Autism, Dyspraxia, A.D.D., Dyslexia, A.D.H.D., Depression, Schizophrenia.* Medinform, 2004.

Capeder, S. *The Four Seasons Diet: Eat Right for Your Season and Lose Weight Effortlessly.* Therapeutae Publishing, 2012.

Food, Inc. (DVD). Directed by Robert Kenner, 2008.

Fresh (DVD). Directed by Ana Sofia Joanes, 2009.

Gottschall, E. *Breaking the Vicious Cycle: Intestinal Health through Diet.* Kirkton Press, 1994.

Hyman, M. *The Blood Sugar Solution: The UltraHealthy Program for Losing Weight, Preventing Disease, and Feeling Great Now!* Little, Brown, 2012.

Lappé, F. M. *Diet for a Small Planet.* Ballantine, 1991.

Linus Pauling Institute, Micronutrient Information Center, http://lpi.oregonstate.edu/infocenter.

Low Dog, T. *Life Is Your Best Medicine: A Woman's Guide to Health, Healing, and Wholeness at Every Age.* National Geographic Society, 2012.

A Place at the Table (DVD). Directed by Kristi Jacobson and Lori Silverbush, 2012.

Pollan, M. *The Omnivore's Dilemma: A Natural History of Four Meals.* Penguin, 2007.

Willett, W. *Eat, Drink, and Be Healthy: The Harvard Medical School Guide to Healthy Eating.* Simon and Schuster, 2005.

Wood, C. *How to Get Kids to Eat Great and Love It: Giving Your Children the Gift of Health with Good Nutrition and Supplementation.* KidsEatGreat, 2002.

Myofascial Disorders, Repetitive Strain Injuries, and Fibromyalgia

"Ergonomics: Human-Centered Design," Cornell University Ergonomics Web, www.ergo.human.cornell.edu.

"Ergonomics and Musculoskeletal Disorders," Centers for Disease Control and Prevention, www.cdc.gov/niosh/topics/ergonomics.

Gunn, C. C. *The Gunn Approach to the Treatment of Chronic Pain: Intramuscular Stimulation for Myofascial Pain of Radiculopathic Origin.* Churchill Livingstone, 1996.

Myers, T. *Anatomy Trains: Myofascial Meridians for Manual and Movement Therapists.* Churchill Livingstone, 2008.

Ober, C., S. Sinatra, and M. Zucker. *Earthing: The Most Important Health Discovery Ever?* Basic Health Publications, 2010.

Pascarelli, E., and D. Quilter. *Repetitive Strain Injury: A Computer User's Guide.* Wiley, 1994.

Putz-Anderson, V., ed. *Cumulative Trauma Disorders: A Manual for Musculoskeletal Diseases of the Upper Limbs.* CRC Press, 1988.

Rolf, I. *Rolfing: Reestablishing the Natural Alignment and Structural Integration of the Human Body for Vitality and Well-Being.* Healing Arts Press, 1989.

"Section A4: Computer Workstations," Princeton University, http://web.princeton.edu /sites/ehs/healthsafetyguide/A4.htm.

Simons, D., and J. Travell. *Myofascial Pain and Dysfunction: The Trigger Point Manual.* Williams and Wilkins, 1998.

Starlanyl, D., and M. E. Copeland. *Fibromyalgia and Chronic Myofascial Pain: A Survival Manual.* New Harbinger, 1997.

Mind-Body Medicine

Borysenko, J. *Minding the Body, Mending the Mind.* Perseus, 2007.

Childre, D. *The HeartMath Solution: The Institute of HeartMath's Revolutionary Program for Engaging the Power of the Heart's Intelligence.* HarperSanFrancisco, 1999.

Chopra, D. *Perfect Health: The Complete Mind/Body Guide.* Random House, 2000.

Dossey, L. *The Extraordinary Healing Power of Ordinary Things: Fourteen Natural Steps to Health and Happiness.* Three Rivers Press, 2006.

Kabat-Zinn, J. *Full Catastrophe Living: Using the Wisdom of Your Body and Mind to Face Stress, Pain and Illness.* Random House, 2005.

————. *Mindfulness Meditation for Pain Relief: Guided Practices for Reclaiming Your Body and Your Life* (audio CD). Sounds True, 2009.

Moyers, B. *Healing and the Mind.* Broadway Books, 1995.

Naparstek, B. *Healing Trauma: Guided Imagery for Posttraumatic Stress* (audio CD). Health Journeys, 1999.

————. *A Meditation for Relaxation and Wellness* (audio CD). Health Journeys, 2002.

————. *Meditations to Relieve Stress* (audio CD). Health Journeys, 1995.

Oz, M. C. *Healing from the Heart: How Unconventional Wisdom Unleashes the Power of Modern Medicine.* Penguin, 1998.

Pert, C. *Molecules of Emotion: The Science behind Mind-Body Medicine.* Simon and Schuster, 1999.

Remen, R. N. *My Grandfather's Blessings: Stories of Strength, Refuge, and Belonging.* Riverhead Books, 2001.

Sapolsky, R. M. *Why Zebras Don't Get Ulcers: The Acclaimed Guide to Stress, Stress-Related Diseases, and Coping.* Henry Holt, 2004.

Exercise

Budilovsky, J., and E. Adamson. *The Complete Idiot's Guide to Yoga.* Alpha, 2006.

Craig, C. *Pilates on the Ball: A Comprehensive Book and DVD Workout.* Healing Arts Press, 2001.

Feldenkrais, M. *Awareness through Movement: Easy-to-Do Health Exercises to Improve Your Posture, Vision, Imagination and Personal Awareness.* HarperCollins, 1990.

Kripalu Yoga: Gentle (DVD). Directed by William Swotes, 2005.

McGee, C., and E. P. Y. Chow. *Miracle Healing from China: Qigong*. MediPress, 1994.

McGonigal, K. *Yoga for Pain Relief: Simple Practices to Calm Your Mind and Heal Your Chronic Pain*. New Harbinger, 2009.

Prudden, B. *Pain Erasure: The Bonnie Prudden Way*. M. Evans, 1980.

Rosenfeld, A. *Tai Chi — The Perfect Exercise: Finding Health, Happiness, Balance, and Strength*. Da Capo, 2013.

Prescription Drugs

Abramson, J. *Overdo$ed America: The Broken Promise of American Medicine*. Harper Perennial, 2005.

Angell, M. *The Truth about Drug Companies: How They Deceive Us and What to Do about It*. Random House, 2005.

Whitaker, R. *The Making of an Epidemic: Magic Bullets, Psychiatric Drugs, and the Astonishing Rise of Mental Illness in America*. Broadway Paperbacks, 2010.

Toxicity

Baker, N. *The Body Toxic: How the Hazardous Chemistry of Everyday Things Threatens Our Health and Well-Being*. North Point Press, 2008.

"EWG's Shopper's Guide to Pesticides in Produce 2013," Environmental Working Group, www.ewg.org/foodnews.

"Guide to Healthy Living," Environmental Working Group, www.ewg.org/guides/cleaners.

"Non-GMO Shopping Guide," www.nongmoshoppingguide.com.

Smith, J. *ShopNoGMO* (phone app). https://itunes.apple.com/us/app/shopnogmo/id646580574?mt=8.

US Environmental Protection Agency website, www.epa.gov.

Wentz, M., and D. Wentz. *The Healthy Home: Simple Truths to Protect Your Family from Hidden Household Dangers*. Vanguard, 2011.

INDEX

rotator cuff tendinitis, 274
running, 152

Sackett, David, 200
SAD (standard American diet), 44,
    239n2 (ch. 4), 240n5
Salford, Leif G., 194–95
salicin, 164
salmonella, 61, 186, 242n23
salt, 140
SAMe (S-adenosylmethionine), 145
saunas, 115
scars, injection of, 218
sciatica, 274
scleroderma, 174
seaweed, 58, 143, 191–92
sedatives, 126–27
seizures, 74
selenium, 242n23
self-care, 119
    healing through, 225–27
    questions about, 228–32
    to-do list, 232–33
Seligman, Martin, 125
Selye, Hans, 245n7
Semi-tough (film; 1977), 265n12
senses, the, 120–21
serotonin, 82, 171, 274
servings, size/number, 56
sex hormones, 168, 176–78
    See also estrogen; testosterone
sexual dysfunction, 171
sexuality, 121, 160
shamanic tradition, 117–18
shock wave therapy, 217
sight, sense of, 120–21
Silent Spring (Carson), 261n7
silymarin, 57, 149, 274
Simons, David G., 237n2, 264n3
Simonton, Carl, 97
Simonton, Karen, 97
Sinatra, Stephen, 212
skin cancer, 114
skin problems, 74
Skootsky, S. A., 263n3
sleep, 130, 131
    dreaming and, 111–12
    habits to encourage, 109
    health benefits of, 106–8

hormone balance and, 176, 178
hours needed, 108–9
IM office visit questions about, 27, 35
interrupted, 110
melatonin produced during, 148
position for, 110–11
sleep medications and, 172
stress hormones and, 259n40
sleep apnea, 107
sleep deprivation, 108, 110, 172
sleep disorders, 88, 110
sleep medications, 54, 172
Slow Food movement, 72
smell, sense of, 120–21
smoke, secondhand, 238n3
smoking, 53, 54, 55
    deaths from, 238n3
    dietary supplements and, 250n18
    health effects of, 105–6, 140
    pain caused by, 171
    quitting, 104–5, 182
snoring, 107
soda, 65, 68–69
sodium, 141
somatic nervous system, 84, 274
somatoemotional release, 210
soy, fermented, 62
specific carbohydrate diet, 76
spelt, 274
spices, 70–71
spinal cord stimulators, 222
spinal injections, 219
spinal surgeries, 222–24
spirituality, 37, 95–96
splints, 213
"standard of care" practices, 11, 159
Staphylococcus aureus, 193, 262–63n27
statins, 19–20, 148, 159–60, 161–62, 172, 182, 275
steroids, 165–67, 218, 220, 256nn13–14, 275
stevia, 65, 275
stomach acid deficiency, 181, 182
stomach problems, 50, 67, 126
stress
    bodily response to, 85–86, 179
    breath during, 90
    emotions and, 87
    identifying, for self-care, 233
    IM office visit discussion of, 27, 32, 36
    inflammation and, 86, 226

ABOUT THE AUTHOR

Heather Tick, MD, has practiced integrative and functional medicine, with an emphasis on integrative pain medicine, for more than twenty years. A leading expert on integrative pain management in the United States and Canada, she has served as director of the Integrative Pain Treatment Center in Toronto, Ontario, since 1993.

Dr. Tick is a clinical associate professor at the University of Washington, in the departments of family medicine and anesthesia and pain medicine. In 2012 she delivered the university's prestigious 27th Gunn-Loke Lecture, and she is the first holder of the Gunn-Loke Endowed Professorship of Integrative Pain Medicine. Dr. Tick served as assistant professor and director of the Integrative Pain Clinic in the department of family and community medicine at the University of Arizona in Tucson; an adjunct professor at the Canadian Memorial Chiropractic College; and a consultant to Heartland Hospice in Tucson, Arizona. She has held teaching positions at the University of Toronto's Wellesley Hospital, at St. Michael's Hospital, and in the department of family medicine at North York General Hospital in Toronto. She is a diplomate of the American Academy of Pain Management, where she served on the education committee.

Dr. Tick is a well-respected researcher in the areas of pain medicine and ergonomics in the workplace. Her articles have been published in *Complementary Therapies in Clinical Practice*, the *American Journal of Physical Medicine and Rehabilitation*, the *Canadian Journal of Rehabilitation*, *Canadian Human Resource Reporter*, and *Hospital News*, and she has written a chapter on integrative pain management for the textbook *Foundations of Pain Medicine and Interventional Pain Management* (ASIPP Publishing, 2011). Her first book, *Life beyond the Carpal Tunnel*, was on repetitive strain injuries.

Dr. Tick also serves as a consultant to corporations — from Fortune 100 companies to small businesses and law firms — regarding ergonomics, health, and safety. She has worked with Accenture, Siemens, Johnson Controls, Keilhauer, Steelcase, the Ontario Ministry of Finance, and *The Globe and Mail*, among other organizations.